Trauma Surgery

S. Di Saverio • G. Tugnoli • F. Catena
L. Ansaloni • N. Naidoo
Editors

Trauma Surgery

Volume 1:
Trauma Management, Trauma Critical Care, Orthopaedic Trauma and Neuro-Trauma

Foreword by Zsolt J. Balogh

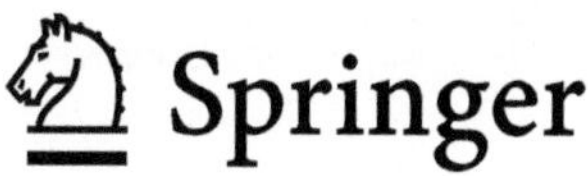

Editors

Salomone Di Saverio
Trauma Surgery Unit
Maggiore Hospital Regional
Trauma Center, AUSL Bologna
Bologna, Italy

Gregorio Tugnoli
Trauma Surgery Unit
Maggiore Hospital Regional
Trauma Center, AUSL Bologna
Bologna, Italy

Fausto Catena
Emergency and Trauma Surgery
Department
Maggiore Hospital of Parma
Parma, Italy

Luca Ansaloni
Department of General
and Emergency Surgery
Papa Giovanni XXIII Hospital
Bergamo, Italy

Noel Naidoo
Department of Surgery
Nelson R Mandela School of Medicine
University of KwaZulu-Natal
Durban, South Africa

Department of Surgery
Port Shepstone Regional Hospital
Durban, South Africa

Videos can also be accessed at http://www.springerimages.com/videos/978-88-470-5403-5

ISBN 978-88-470-5402-8   ISBN 978-88-470-5403-5   (eBook)
DOI 10.1007/978-88-470-5403-5
Springer Milan Heidelberg New York Dordrecht London

Library of Congress Control Number: 2013951145

© Springer-Verlag Italia 2014
This work is subject to copyright. All rights are reserved by the Publisher, whether the whole or part of the material is concerned, specifically the rights of translation, reprinting, reuse of illustrations, recitation, broadcasting, reproduction on microfilms or in any other physical way, and transmission or information storage and retrieval, electronic adaptation, computer software, or by similar or dissimilar methodology now known or hereafter developed. Exempted from this legal reservation are brief excerpts in connection with reviews or scholarly analysis or material supplied specifically for the purpose of being entered and executed on a computer system, for exclusive use by the purchaser of the work. Duplication of this publication or parts thereof is permitted only under the provisions of the Copyright Law of the Publisher's location, in its current version, and permission for use must always be obtained from Springer. Permissions for use may be obtained through RightsLink at the Copyright Clearance Center. Violations are liable to prosecution under the respective Copyright Law.
The use of general descriptive names, registered names, trademarks, service marks, etc. in this publication does not imply, even in the absence of a specific statement, that such names are exempt from the relevant protective laws and regulations and therefore free for general use.
While the advice and information in this book are believed to be true and accurate at the date of publication, neither the authors nor the editors nor the publisher can accept any legal responsibility for any errors or omissions that may be made. The publisher makes no warranty, express or implied, with respect to the material contained herein.

Printed on acid-free paper

Springer is part of Springer Science+Business Media (www.springer.com)

With deep gratitude I'd like to dedicate this work to the memory of my father, Tito, who recognized my inclinations early on, encouraged and supported me with wonderful enthusiasm and intelligence in my pursuit of a medical and surgical career. His constant presence in my youth, his optimism, his simple and honest life are for me still a source of pride and a never ending model for life, being a star from the sky, shining brightly to give me a safe and fatherly guidance!

I also thank and dedicate to my mother, Gabriella, who has always been the beacon of light guiding me morally and culturally. She is a brilliant combination of religious faith and classical learning who supported me in my commitment to research and science. She remains my mentor in logic and humanities, sharing the wisdom of her beloved Greek and Latin masters.

I am also grateful and dedicate to my devoted wife Omeshnie from South Africa, a professional nurse whom I met during my experience overseas as a trauma surgeon. She constantly supports me and every day she is sharing our life together with patience and love.

Salomone

To my mum and dad, for all they have done for me.

To Luisa, Francesca and Alessandro, with all my love.

To my young grandson Federico, with my best wishes for his future life.

Gregorio

To all world Emergency Surgeons: brave and good people

Fausto

Trauma Vol 1: To my beautiful and amazing wife Claudia and my family
Trauma Vol 2: To my amazing parents Gina and Atchiah Naidoo and my family

Noel

Foreword

It is a pleasure to see the result of the Italian group of editors' (Di Saverio, Tugnoli, Catena, Ansaloni and Naidoo) exemplary effort to produce a landmark textbook about trauma care. They have pulled together the best of the academic trauma brother-/sisterhood and well beyond to make this book as primarily an "Italian job" considering many world leaders among the authors practice on the Apennine Peninsula or have an ancestral claim there. Italy and Italian Trauma Care needs this fine example of a documented, well-organised approach for the further development of their trauma system and the recognition of trauma as a specialty within surgery and critical care.

It is a common phrase that trauma is a leading cause of death and long term disability in the young, productive age groups. While this is still true, we need to acknowledge the enormous advances in polytrauma management during the last decades. Major trauma mortality in trauma centres is half of the figures compared to the mortality 20 years ago. This is even more significant in the context of the currently treated trauma population who tend to be slightly more severely injured but on average at least 10 years older. The overall trauma mortality in developed level-1 trauma centres is less than 3 % of all admissions and less than 9 % counting only the patients with injury severity score higher than 15. Trauma mortality review panels hardly find preventable trauma deaths in the developed trauma systems. These facts force us to look for clinically more relevant and improvable outcomes beyond the plummeting mortality, such as resource utilisation (~quaternary prevention) and quality of life among the survivors.

Volume 1 of the *Trauma Surgery* textbook addresses some of the most important contributors of these outcomes (trauma systems, critical care, head injury and musculoskeletal trauma). Trauma system and head injury management remain the key determinants of mortality; head injury is still the leading cause of death in most geographic areas and organised trauma system/program has the biggest impact on the reduction of trauma mortality.

Critical care including perioperative polytrauma management (initial resuscitation, damage control surgery, postoperative ongoing ICU care) is the most resource intensive component of the hospital phase. Optimal management recommended in this book is essential to prevent deadly and expensive complications such as thromboembolic disease, infections, organ dysfunctions and multiple organ failure.

Musculoskeletal injuries including spine and pelvis are the most frequently operated on injuries; especially in blunt trauma, their optimal timing and methods of stabilisation are still commonly debated topics. It is concluded that these, not necessarily always life threatening injuries, are the major determinants of the functional outcome. This is relevant both to the survivors of major trauma and to the isolated limb injury patients. Suboptimal outcomes of these injuries result in long term or permanent disability, which is a major psychosocial and financial burden on the injured patient and on the entire society.

Hopefully this book will promote the knowledge necessary to manage these complex patients through generations of trauma surgeons and other clinicians committed to the multidisciplinary management of the injured.

Zsolt J. Balogh
MD, PhD, FRACS(Ortho), FAOrthA, FACS
John Hunter Hospital and University of Newcastle
Newcastle, NSW, Australia

Preface

When in the summer of 2011 our small group of Acute Care and Trauma Surgeons, founder members of World Society of Emergency Surgery, had a joined meeting, we all together felt there was a strong need for improving education in the field of acute care and trauma surgery, especially for younger surgeons, or any doctor or professional, approaching for the first time this discipline and the complex management of trauma patients. This need is even stronger in these days, when the decreased surgical training opportunities, combined with the changes in epidemiology and severity of Trauma as well as the spreading use of Non-Operative management, all these have been factors contributing to make the career of a Trauma Surgeon a field of "missed opportunities". This is more evident if compared to the role that Trauma Sugery had in the past decades, when it has definitely had a unique and peerless educational value. In the last decades, in fact, a "good performing" general surgeon would have never missed during his training a valuable experience in a trauma surgery service.

We have therefore had the idea of writing a book of trauma surgery, aiming to offer a practical manual of procedures, techniques and operative strategies, rather than pretending to be an excessively long, perhaps excruciating, textbook of trauma surgery.

Our book should have had the form of an handbook, offering a fresh overview of operative techniques and management strategies in trauma for the general surgeon, for the resident/trainee, for any surgeon who is not dealing everyday with trauma case and for any professional (even scrub nurses) involved in the care of traumatized patient who wants to have a clear and practical idea of what should be quickly and effectively done in the Operating Room in case of a major trauma. A modern trauma surgeon should know how to repair multiple traumatic injuries, which may occur in different body regions, how to perfom the needed procedures in the best sequence possible, both giving the correct priority to every action and gaining the most convenient access for the best anatomic exposure. Furthermore he must be inspired to the concepts of damage control and should be competent in controlling hemorrhage and contamination quickly, and in discerning when to end surgery and send the patient to ICU and/or angio-suite.

After more than a year of hard work, it is now with great pleasure that we are announcing the completion of our ambitious project of a trauma surgery manual, where most of the renowned trauma surgeons from all over the world have made an appreciable and highly valuable contribution, with the intent not to merely describe in academic fashion the most recent surgical techniques, but rather to suggest the best surgical strategies in terms of keeping things simple but effective when in OR, and sharing their expertise for achieving a wise clinical judgment and good common sense. We hope this manual may represent a true "vademecum" with the specific aim of giving a fresh view and practical suggestions for the best management of trauma and improving the skills of the treating surgeons.

Once again I would like to thankfully acknowledge the excellent level of scientific quality and educational value of the content that each chapter's author have contributed.

The material received was so extensive in terms of quantity and quality that the contents have been apportioned between two volumes. The first regarding Trauma Management, Critical Care, Orthopedic Trauma and Neuro-Trauma and the second including Thoracic and Abdominal Trauma.

We are moreover very glad that this project, conducted in cooperation with our World Society of Emergency Surgery and its Journal, has truly joined together trauma surgeons from all over the world sharing our experiences in trauma. The multidisciplinary board of authors, editors and foreword writers of this book is truly International with contributors from the Americas (USA, Canada, Brazil, Argentina), Europe (Italy, Germany, Finland, Austria, France, UK, Turkey), Africa (South Africa), Australasia (Australia and New Zealand), and Asia (Israel, Turkey, India). This is a most heartening and promising signal for the future of our discipline worldwide, demonstrating that Trauma Surgery remains a vibrant surgical discipline.

This is the first of further planned WSES Books, promising to be the starting cornerstone of the WSES Educational Program for the next future years. This project aims to link together WSES Courses, WSES Guidelines and WSES Books to give complete educational tools to the next generation of emergency and trauma surgeons. We are aiming to proceed shortly with the WSES acute care surgery book.

I would also like to acknowledge the invaluable foreword contributions from Dr. K. Mattox, Dr. F. Baldoni, Dr. C. W. Schwab and Dr. K. Brohi, emanating from their extensive experiences.

Finally, a special thanks and a debt of gratitude to the Springer team who worked tirelessly over this period with unwavering professionalism, in particular Alessandra Born and Donatella Rizza. Without them this publication would not have been made possible, and it reinforces Springer's value and position as the leading publisher in medical education.

We look forward to a successful and well received set of publications and a worldwide ongoing cooperation within our international family of enthusiastic trauma surgeons.

Bologna, Italy   Dr. Salomone Di Saverio, MD

co-editors

Bologna, Italy   Dr. Gregorio Tugnoli, MD
Bologna, Italy   Dr. Fausto Catena, MD
Bologna, Italy   Dr. Luca Ansaloni, MD
Johannesburg, South Africa   Dr. Noel Naidoo, MD

Contents

1 Training, Education, and Decision-Making in Trauma Surgery 1
Hee Soo Jung and Lena M. Napolitano

2 Management of the Polytrauma Patient 17
David J.J. Muckart and Noel Naidoo

3 Damage Control Resuscitation 27
Juan Carlos Duchesne, Bruno Monteiro Pereira, and Gustavo Pereira Fraga

4 Principles and Philosophy of Damage Control Surgery. 43
Fredric M. Pieracci and Ernest E. Moore

5 Surgical Treatment of Pelvic Fractures. 65
Raffaele Pascarella, Luigi Rizzi, Claudio Castelli, and Rocco Politano

6 Surgery of the Cervical Spine Trauma 73
Federico De Iure and Luca Amendola

7 Surgery of the Thoracolumbar Spine Trauma 81
Ralf H. Gahr and Mathias Spalteholz

8   Trauma Surgery of the Extremities   89
Ralf H. Gahr and Matthias Spalteholz

**9   Minimally Invasive Approach and Endovascular
Techniques for Vascular Trauma**   109
Joseph J. DuBose, Megan Brenner,
and Thomas M. Scalea

**10   Interventional Techniques for Hemorrhage
Control in Trauma**   121
Robert Short, Alan Murdock, Phillip Orons,
and Andrew B. Peitzman

11   Management of Penetrating Neck Injuries   149
Patrizio Petrone, Juan M. Verde,
and Juan A. Asensio

**12   Acute Traumatic Brain Injuries and Their
Management**   165
Michael M. Krausz, Itamar Ashkenazi,
and Jean F. Soustiel

13   Establishing a Trauma Service   183
David J.J. Muckart and Noel Naidoo

14   Multiple Organ Failure in Trauma Patients   191
Francesco Del Corso, Carlo Coniglio,
Aimone Giugni, Francesca Mengoli,
Francesco Boni, Ilaria Turriziani, Gregorio Tugnoli,
Salomone Di Saverio, and Giovanni Gordini

15   Infections in Trauma Patients   205
Massimo Sartelli and Cristian Tranà

Chapter 1
Training, Education, and Decision-Making in Trauma Surgery

Hee Soo Jung and Lena M. Napolitano

1.1 Introduction

Trauma is a heavy burden to healthcare worldwide. In 2011, accidental injury accounted for over 120,000 deaths and was the fifth largest cause of death in the United States (USA) [1]. There were also over 54,000 deaths related to intentional self-harm and assault [1]. In the European Union (EU), 15 % of deaths

H.S. Jung, MD
Surgical Critical Care, Surgery Department,
University of Michigan Health System,
Room 1C340-UH, University Hospital,
1500 East Medical Drive, SPC 5033, Ann Arbor, MI 48104, USA
e-mail: heesooj@umich.edu

L.M. Napolitano, MD, FACS, FCCP, FCCM (⊠)
Division of Acute Care Surgery,
Trauma, Burn, Critical Care, Emergency Surgery,
University of Michigan Health System,
Room 1C340-UH, University Hospital,
1500 East Medical Center Drive, SPC 5033,
Ann Arbor, MI 48109-5033, USA
e-mail: lenan@umich.edu

S. Di Saverio et al. (eds.), *Trauma Surgery*,
DOI 10.1007/978-88-470-5403-5_1, © Springer-Verlag Italia 2014

before age 60 are related to injuries [2]. Similarly worldwide, an estimated five million deaths are attributed to injuries each year with about 70 % related to unintentional injuries and 30 % related to intentional injuries [3].

1.2 History of Trauma Surgery

While the treatment of injury has a long history in medicine, the establishment of trauma systems and the organization of trauma training are relatively new. In the USA, the first trauma centers opened in the 1960s. Statewide and national regionalization of trauma care occurred shortly thereafter [4]. In 1978, the Advanced Trauma Life Support (ATLS) program was introduced in Nebraska to offer consensus views on approaches to early trauma management and to provide organized training for physicians providers [5]. Modeled after the successful Advanced Cardiac Life Support (ACLS) program, ATLS was the first in standardized national trauma training and has recently published its 9th edition (October 2012).

ATLS was adopted by the American College of Surgeons (ACS) and developed into an international course that has trained over one million participants in over 50 countries [5]. It is the longest standing and most widely adopted trauma course in the world. ATLS has become the foundation of care for injured patients by teaching a common language and a common approach to trauma care in the global community.

Optimal worldwide trauma care is the ultimate goal. Defining the resources necessary to assure such care in all regions is challenging. In 2004, the World Health Organization (WHO) published Guidelines for Essential Trauma Care to set achievable standards for trauma treatment services which could realistically be made available to almost every injured person worldwide [6].

1.3   Fundamental Competencies of a Trauma Surgeon

The areas that a trauma surgeon must master are expansive. Injuries occur across all organ systems, and the knowledge needed to treat each patient is both broad and detailed. Trauma surgeons must often rapidly process evolving data about the patient's injury and condition. There are many diagnostic and therapeutic skills that a trauma surgeon must be facile in. The ability to quickly and independently interpret the physical exam, laboratory studies, and imaging findings is crucial to rapid treatment. Surgeons are expected to be able to rapidly obtain airway control and intravenous access and perform lifesaving interventions such as tube thoracostomies and resuscitative thoracotomies.

Trauma operative care is also complex. It can involve multiple organs and body compartments in physiologically altered patients. This difficulty is compounded because diagnosis is often unknown while the planning phase must be by nature brief but thorough. The trauma surgeon also concurrently provides real-time critical care—treating shock and organ failure.

Furthermore, this work must all be performed within the context of a difficult environment. Trauma care is time sensitive. One must take quick action regarding the problem at hand while taking into account the various hidden pitfalls that could be lurking around the corner. Surgeons must be able to be detail oriented while not losing situational awareness and efficiency. They are often placed in leadership roles in large teams consisting of many types of healthcare personnel and complex relationships. They must be effective while coordinating care with many consultants and across different hospital settings. Expertise in healthcare systems and the ability to triage patients and manage finite resources is required. Vulnerabilities and limitations within the trauma system, the trauma care team, and the trauma surgeon must be recognized and planned for.

1.4 Current Status of Trauma Training

1.4.1 Graduate Medical Education

In the USA, trauma surgeons first complete a 5-year general surgery residency after undergraduate medical education. Trauma surgery is formally incorporated into general surgical residency education. There is a minimum requirement of 10 operative trauma cases, 20 nonoperative trauma cases, and 25 surgical critical care cases. In 2012, graduating residents averaged 29 operative trauma and 48 nonoperative trauma cases [7]. To obtain board certification in general surgery, certification must also be obtained in ATLS and ACLS [8].

Most practicing trauma surgeons also obtain board certification in surgical critical care through a 1-year ACGME-approved fellowship. This is sometimes associated with an additional year in trauma or acute care surgery. There is currently no separate board certification for trauma surgery. The American Association for the Surgery of Trauma (AAST) has begun to standardize and approve Acute Care Surgery programs, providing a certification of completion from the AAST. Fellowships in Acute Care Surgery are 2 years in duration (1 year surgical critical care, 1 year acute care surgery, including training in emergency general surgery and surgical subspecialties). Acute Care Surgery fellowships are replacing many trauma fellowship positions in the USA [9].

Data suggests that current US training pathways, especially those that include a second trauma year, are sufficient in training trauma surgeons [10]. However, there is also evidence to suggest that several years of postgraduate experience in practice is required for new trauma surgeons to obtain similar outcomes to more experienced surgeons [11]. This is not surprising given the unpredictable nature of the disease processes and need for quick expert decisions.

While European surgical training is more heterogeneous, the European Board of Surgery has similar requirements for the training of trauma surgeons. The minimum acceptable duration of training for European Board of Surgery Qualification in Trauma Surgery is 7 years [12]. This must include a minimum of 5 years in specialist surgical units for common trunk training. Candidates must have completed 2 years training in a Trauma Unit and must provide documentation of a specific number of surgical procedures in trauma, serving as principal surgeon or first assistant.

1.4.2   Trauma Education and Training Programs

There are a number of trauma didactic programs available both nationally and internationally for the education of trauma team providers (Table 1.1).

Table 1.1 List of trauma educational resources

Trauma courses
Advanced Trauma Life Support (ATLS)
http://www.facs.org/trauma/atls/about.html
Trauma Evaluation and Management (TEAM) for medical students
http://www.facs.org/trauma/atls/team.html
Advanced Trauma Care for Nurses (ATCN) for registered nurses
http://www.traumanurses.org/atcn-courses.html
PreHospital Trauma Life Support (PHTLS) for prehospital care providers
http://www.naemt.org/education/PHTLS/phtls.aspx
Definitive Perioperative Nurses Trauma Care Course (DPNTC)
http://www.dstc.co.nz/
Trauma Nurse Core Course (TNCC)
http://www.ena.org/coursesandeducation/ENPC-TNCC/tncc/Pages/aboutcourse.aspx
International Trauma Life Support (ITLS) for prehospital trauma care
http://www.itrauma.org/resources/ITLSeTrauma.asp

1.4.2.1 Advanced Trauma Life Support (ATLS)

ATLS is now in its 9th edition, published October 2012. It is now an international course that has been adapted successfully in many different settings, providing a common language for trauma training that can save lives in critical situations. ATLS teaches a systematic, concise approach to the early management of trauma patients. It is available to physicians in the different fields that provide trauma care. The focus is on standardized and systematic approaches. The primary and secondary surveys are used as a framework with cues to prioritize life-threatening issues as they are recognized. The course includes didactics and practical sessions. Testing includes a written exam and simulated scenarios.

The 9th edition of ATLS includes a number of new content updates (Table 1.2). It now offers mobile content (MyATLS) as a point-of-care reference. Clinicians can use the MyATLS app on smartphones or tablets to access and use critical references and resources regarding trauma care at the patient's bedside or in the field. Videos and animations review key trauma skills. Algorithms, calculators, and formulas put lifesaving trauma information at the fingertips of the primary trauma providers.

Table 1.2 Advanced Trauma Life Support (ATLS) 9th Edition—content updates

Concept of balanced resuscitation
Emphasis on the pelvis as a source of blood loss
Use of more advanced airway techniques for the difficult airway
Optional DPL and pericardiocentesis
New FAST skill station
New multiple-choice questions for pretest and posttest
Optional expanded content on heat injury
New initial assessment scenarios
Many new images
New Instructor Course content
New skills videos
New ATLS App (MyATLS)

1.4.2.2 Trauma Evaluation and Management (TEAM)

The TEAM course is offered at the undergraduate medical education level and also serves as an educational resource for other trauma team members. It is an abbreviated version of ATLS designed to teach basic trauma assessment and management. This serves as an introduction for further ATLS training.

1.4.2.3 Trauma Surgical Skills Courses

To manage trauma competently, there is a need to master operative skills that cover the abdominal cavity (including the pelvis and retroperitoneum), the thorax and mediastinum, and the peripheral vascular system. In particular, the rapid exposure required to control traumatic bleeding is a mandatory skill for the trauma surgeon.

The acquisition of these definitive surgical trauma skills for our general surgical residents is difficult in our current era of increasing nonoperative management of blunt traumatic injuries [13–16]. With the decline in operative cases in trauma surgery, operative skills training courses have become important adjuncts to trauma training. There are several courses that teach operative management and surgical skills in trauma (Table 1.3). For general surgery residency programs with challenges in providing adequate clinical exposure to operative trauma management in their institutions, it is recommended that program directors consider specific operative skills training courses that can meet the requirements of this specific training need and also provide an objective competency assessment. These operative skills training courses should be considered for senior surgical residents at the level of postgraduate year 4 or higher. The ACGME endorses the concept of evaluation of (1) individual milestones and (2) assessment of objective measures of operative skills in the general surgery residency curriculum. These trauma surgical skills courses can assist in achieving these objectives.

Table 1.3 Trauma surgical skills courses

1. *ATOM – Advanced Trauma Operative Management*
    (a) The ATOM course is an effective method of increasing surgical competence in the operative management of penetrating injuries to the chest and abdomen and is provided by the American College of Surgeons Committee on Trauma
    (b) Information: http://atomcourse.com/about.php
    (c) Find a course: http://atomcourse.com/find.php
2. *ASSET – Advanced Surgical Skills for Exposure in Trauma*
    (a) The ASSET course uses human cadavers to teach surgical exposure of anatomic structures that when injured may pose a threat to life or limb
    (b) Information: http://www.facs.org/trauma/education/asset.html
    (c) Find a course: http://www.facs.org/trauma/education/assetcourse.html
3. *DSTS – Definitive Surgical Trauma Skills*
    (a) The DSTS course is a 2-day hands-on practical cadaveric workshop course developed by the Royal College of Surgeons of England with the Royal Defence Medical College and the Uniformed Services University of the Health Sciences in the USA
    (b) Information: http://www.rcseng.ac.uk/education/courses/ surgical_trauma.html
4. *DSTC – Definitive Surgical Trauma Care*
    (a) The Definitive Surgical Trauma Care (DSTC) 2-day course focuses on surgical decision-making and surgical operative technique in critically ill trauma patients. It was developed by the International Association for Trauma and Surgical Intensive Care (IATSIC) of the International Surgical Society and is recommended by the Royal Australian College of Surgeons for all surgeons involved in the management of major trauma
    (b) Information: http://www.dstc.co.nz/
5. *Other institution-based trauma operative skills courses*:
    (a) *Trauma Exposure Course (TEC)* – 1-day 8-h structured skills curriculum course using fresh cadavers which focuses on operative exposure of human anatomic structures in the neck, chest, abdomen, and extremities. Developed at University of Texas Southwestern Medical Center, Dallas, TX. (See Gunst et al. [19])

Advanced Trauma Operative Management (ATOM) is a 1-day course offered by ACS to provide training in the operative management of penetrating injuries to the chest and abdomen [17]. It utilizes standardized didactics, audiovisual aids, and porcine model simulation to train surgeons in these techniques. The ACS Advanced Surgical Skills for Exposure in Trauma (ASSET) course, the Royal College of Surgeons of England Definitive Surgical Trauma Skills course, and the University of Texas Trauma Exposure Course (TEC) are examples of similar hands-on workshop courses that teach operative trauma skills on human cadaveric models [18–20].

As new surgical techniques are developed for use in trauma care, new interactive and skills-based educational programs will be established to supplement training. An example is training for endovascular trauma interventions, including resuscitative balloon occlusion of the aorta [21]. Currently, the Endovascular Skills for Trauma and Resuscitative Surgery course [22], a joint military-civilian educational effort, is in the process of refinement and validation. This course targets practicing trauma surgeons who desire to gain knowledge and skills in endovascular treatment of traumatic injuries.

1.4.3 Training in Underdeveloped Trauma Systems

Different countries and regions have different situations, resources, and needs that might not be served as well by trauma training programs developed for mature trauma systems [6, 23]. The WHO Guidelines for Essential Trauma Care defines basic physician/provider training requirements needed for establishing trauma care systems worldwide [6].

The International Association for Trauma and Surgical Intensive Care (IATSIC) has developed two courses with the specific circumstances of lower resource countries in mind [6]. The National Trauma Management Course (NMTC), developed in India, is a 2-day course focused on early trauma management similar to the ATLS program. The Definitive Surgical Trauma Course (DSTC) is a program similar to the ATOM and ASSET courses and also includes a cadaver or animal model component. It is targeted for surgeons and teaches operative management of difficult traumatic injuries.

1.5 Educational Methods and Resources

1.5.1 Books

The Surgical Council on Resident Education (SCORE) curriculum has become the standard for general surgery residency training in the USA (https://portal.surgicalcore.org/). The SCORE general surgery resident curriculum has established uniform learning objectives, compiled text references and video resources, and offers knowledge assessments for general surgery residents. It contains an extensive section on trauma and is an important resource especially for surgical residents in the USA.

Most standard textbooks of surgery contain a significant section on trauma. There are also several excellent textbooks which focus on the care of the trauma patient. Institutional trauma handbooks play a similar but important role. They define the local protocols that are crucial in the management of trauma patients on a day-to-day basis.

There are also well-regarded reference works that deal more specifically with decision-making processes in trauma surgery. These include *Top Knife* [24], a book which delves into the various nuances of operative trauma strategies, and a 2007 review on pitfalls in trauma management [25].

1.5.2 Algorithms, Guidelines, and Protocols

Evidence-based protocols, guidelines, and algorithms are vital components to trauma patient care and trauma education. Recently, guideline compliance in trauma by the implementation of standard operating procedures has been documented in two important prospective randomized studies to significantly improve trauma outcomes [26–28].

Institutions providing trauma care must adapt national algorithms and guidelines into protocols for use within their own institutions. While not perfect in every situation, management algorithms and guidelines are important tools that allow us to quickly apply known scientific data to relevant patient care problems. The Eastern Association for the Surgery of Trauma provides practice management guidelines which systematically review the evidence and make recommendations for optimal trauma management [29]. The Western Trauma Association publishes algorithms which allows guideline implementation by providing step-by-step processes for clinical decision-making [30]. Other societies such as the Society of Critical Care Medicine also provide guidelines related to trauma care. While algorithms and protocols must be adapted for individual patient circumstances, they provide a framework from which effective evidence-based clinical action can be taken (Table 1.4).

Table 1.4 Guidelines and algorithms in trauma care

Eastern Association for the Surgery of Trauma (EAST) Practice Management Guidelines

http://www.east.org/resources/treatment-guidelines

Western Trauma Association (WTA) Algorithms

http://westerntrauma.org/algorithms/algorithms.html

Society of Critical Care Medicine (SCCM) Guidelines

http://www.learnicu.org/Pages/Guidelines.aspx

1.6 Trauma Performance Improvement

As in all of medicine, critical appraisal of individual and system performance is necessary to provide optimal trauma patient care. There are several methods by which this can be undertaken.

1.6.1 Simulation Training and Video Review

Trauma situations are high-stake situations. While direct patient care can add important teaching moments, additional learning environments have been sought. High-fidelity human patient simulators have been shown to be effective practice models for trauma scenarios. They have been shown to improve teamwork and communication, decision-making, efficiency, and self-confidence while decreasing adverse outcomes [31–33]. These can be combined with video review and debriefing which can efficiently detect performance errors and further improve performance [34, 35].

1.6.2 Case Logs

Individual case logs allow surgeons to track the breadth and volume of their clinical experience. It also allows one to identify complications and unexpected outcomes. It provides a framework for later performance improvement and research efforts. Many case log systems exist, including the ACS Case Log System.

1.6.3 Trauma Quality Improvement Program (TQIP)

Quality improvement programs offer a practical means to achieve improvements in trauma care and are the trauma system equivalent of individual case logs. These programs enable trauma providers and healthcare institutions to better monitor their trauma care services and outcomes, detect problems, and enact and evaluate corrective measures. This is accomplished at the patient, institutional, state, and national level. To give guidance in this area, the World Health Organization released "Guidelines for Trauma Quality Improvement Programmes" in June 2009. The guidelines review the most common methods of quality improvement in trauma care in a how-to-do fashion, covering a wide range of techniques intended to be universally applicable to all countries [36].

An example of a mature national quality improvement program is the ACS TQIP [37] which utilizes the infrastructure of the National Trauma Data Bank [38]. Similar to the ACS National Surgical Quality Improvement Program (NSQIP), TQIP offers validated, risk-adjusted benchmarking for accurate feedback to institutions regarding trauma care. It also identifies institutional characteristics which are associated with improved trauma outcomes. ACS TQIP currently has over 160 participating trauma centers in the USA. Regional and statewide trauma quality improvement programs or collaboratives are also very effective in improving trauma care regionally [39].

1.7 Conclusion

As complex and rewarding as the practice of trauma surgery is, the preparation required to master it successfully is equally multifaceted and extensive and requires appropriate training and education. Trauma surgery education has advanced significantly in the last decade, with the advent of didactic and operative skills training courses, high-fidelity patient simulator and team training, evidence-based algorithms, guidelines and protocols, and trauma performance improvement programs. Optimal trauma surgery education and training can prepare a surgeon to proficiently treat critically injured patients and provides trauma surgeons with the knowledge and confidence to act swiftly and purposefully in treating the patient with life-threatening injuries.

References

1. Hoyert DL, Xu J (2012) Deaths: preliminary data for 2011. Natl Vital Stat Rep 61(6):40–42
2. Zimmermann N, Bauer R (2006) Injuries in the European Union: Statistics summary 2002–2004: European Commission/Health and Consumer Protection (DG Sanco)
3. Roux D, Ricard J-D (2011) Novel therapies for Pseudomonas aeruginosa pneumonia. Infect Disord Drug Targets 11(4):389–394
4. Boyd DR (2010) Trauma systems origins in the United States. J Trauma Nurs 17(3):126–135
5. Kortbeek JB et al (2008) Advanced trauma life support, 8th edition, the evidence for change. J Trauma 64:1638–1650
6. Mock C, Lormand JD, Goosen J, Joshipura M, Peden M (2004) Guidelines for Essential Trauma Care. World Health Organization, Geneva. http://whqlibdoc.who.int/publications/2004/9241546409.pdf. Accessed 2013
7. Celik IH, Oguz SS, Demirel G, Erdeve O, Dilmen U (2012) Outcome of ventilator-associated pneumonia due to multidrug-resistant Acinetobacter baumannii and Pseudomonas aeruginosa treated with aerosolized colistin in neonates: a retrospective chart review. Eur J Pediatr 171(2):311–316
8. The American Board of Surgery. Booklet of Information, Surgery, 2012–2013. http://home.absurgery.org/xfer/BookletofInfo-Surgery.pdf. Accessed 2013
9. Napolitano LM et al (2010) Challenging issues in surgical critical care, trauma, and acute care surgery: a report from the Critical Care Committee of the American Association for the Surgery of Trauma. J Trauma 69(6):1619–1633
10. Reilly PM et al (2003) Training in trauma surgery: quantitative and qualitative aspects of a new paradigm for fellowship. Ann Surg 238(4):596–604
11. McKenney MG et al (2009) Trauma surgeon mortality rates correlate with surgeon time at institution. J Am Coll Surg 208:750–754

12. Syllabus in trauma surgery. http://www.uemssurg.org: European Board of Surgery, Division of Traumatology. Accessed 2012
13. Drake FT et al (2012) ACGME case logs: surgery resident experience in operative trauma for two decades. J Trauma Acute Care Surg 73(6):1498–1504
14. Bulinski P et al (2003) The changing face of trauma management and its impact on surgical resident training. J Trauma 54(1):161–163
15. Fakhry SM et al (2003) The resident experience on trauma: declining surgical opportunities and career incentives? Analysis of data from large multi-institutional study. J Trauma 54(1):1–8
16. Bittner JG IV et al (2010) Nonoperative management of solid organ injury diminishes surgical resident operative experience: is it time for simulation training? J Surg Res 163:179–185
17. Jacobs LM et al (2006) Advanced trauma operative management course: site and instructor selection and evaluation. J Am Coll Surg 203(5):772–779
18. Ali J et al (2011) Potential role for the Advanced Surgical Skills for Exposure in Trauma (ASSET) course in Canada. J Trauma 71(6):1491–1493
19. Gunst M et al (2009) Trauma operative skills in the era of nonoperative management: the trauma exposure course (TEC). J Trauma 67(5):1091–1096
20. Ryan JM, Roberts P (2002) Definitive surgical trauma skills: a new skills course for specialist registrars and consultants in general surgery in the United Kingdom. Trauma 4:184–188
21. Stannard A et al (2011) Resuscitative endovascular balloon occlusion of the aorta (REBOA) as an adjunct for hemorrhagic shock. J Trauma 71(6):1869–1872
22. Rasmussen TE et al (2011) Vascular trauma at a crossroads. J Trauma 70(5):1291–1293
23. Drimousis PG et al (2011) Advanced Trauma Life Support certifies physician in a non trauma system setting: Is it enough? Resuscitation 82:180–184
24. Hirschberg A, Mattox KL (2005) Top knife: the art & craft of trauma surgery. tfm Publishing, Shrewsbury
25. Mackersie RC (2007) Pitfalls in the evaluation and management of the trauma patient. Curr Probl Surg 44:778–833
26. Napolitano LM (2012) Guideline compliance in trauma: evidence-based protocols to improve trauma outcomes? Crit Care Med 40(3):990–992
27. Rice TW et al (2012) Deviations from evidence-based clinical management guidelines increase mortality in critically injured trauma patients. Crit Care Med 40(3):778–786

28. Cuschieri J et al (2012) Benchmarking outcomes in the critically injured trauma patient and the effect of implementing standard operating procedures. Ann Surg 255(5):993–999
29. Eastern Association for the Surgery of Trauma Practice Management Guidelines. http://www.east.org/resources/treatment-guidelines. Accessed 2012
30. McIntyre R Jr et al (2012) Western Trauma Association algorithms. http://westerntrauma.org/algorithms/algorithms.html. Accessed 2012
31. Holcomb JB et al (2002) Evaluation of trauma team performance using an advanced human patient simulator for resuscitation training. J Trauma 52(6):1078–1085
32. Marshall RL et al (2001) Use of a human patient simulator in the development of resident trauma management skills. J Trauma 51(1):17–21
33. Capella J et al (2010) Teamwork training improves the clinical care of trauma patients. J Surg Educ 67(6):439–443
34. Hamilton NA et al (2012) Video review using a reliable evaluation metric improves team function in high-fidelity simulated trauma resuscitation. J Surg Educ 69(3):428–431
35. Georgiou A, Lockey DJ (2010) The performance and assessment of hospital trauma teams. Scand J Trauma Resusc Emerg Med 18:66
36. Mock C, Juillard C, Brundage S, Goosen J, Joshipura M (2009) Guidelines for trauma quality improvement programmes. World Health Organization, Geneva. http://whqlibdoc.who.int/publications/2009/9789241597746_eng.pdf. Accessed 2013
37. American College of Surgeons Trauma Quality Improvement Program. http://www.facs.org/trauma/ntdb/tqip.html. Accessed 2012
38. American College of Surgeons National Trauma Data Bank. http://www.facs.org/trauma/ntdb/index.html. Accessed 2012
39. Michigan Trauma Quality Improvement Program. http://www.mtqip.org/. Accessed 2012

Chapter 2
Management of the Polytrauma Patient

David J.J. Muckart and Noel Naidoo

Traumatic brain injury (TBI) and hemorrhage account for the vast majority of early trauma deaths [1], the latter contributing to severe secondary brain injury. Primary TBI is irreversible, whereas the effects of hemorrhage on both cerebral and other body systems may be countered by aggressive and appropriate resuscitation which is the first critical step when managing polytrauma. The goal of resuscitation is to normalize oxygen delivery (DO_2) and oxygen consumption (VO_2) and restore aerobic metabolism. Thereafter, the management consists of identifying injuries, prioritizing surgical management, and preventing or supporting organ dysfunction.

The switch from anaerobic to aerobic metabolism is a crucial goal and is underscored by a few simple biochemical facts. Adenosine triphosphate (ATP) is virtually the sole energy source for the myriad of life-sustaining human cellular reactions

D.J.J. Muckart, FRCS, MMedSci (✉) • N. Naidoo, FCS (SA)
Department of Surgery, Nelson R Mandela School of Medicine,
University of KwaZulu-Natal, 719 Umbilo Road,
Durban, Republic of South Africa
e-mail: davidmuc@ialch.co.za; noel.naidoo@gmail.com

S. Di Saverio et al. (eds.), *Trauma Surgery*,
DOI 10.1007/978-88-470-5403-5_2, © Springer-Verlag Italia 2014

and is produced during oxidative phosphorylation within the mitochondria by Krebs cycle. At any one time the body contains only 100 g of ATP, yet the average daily requirements are between 100 and 150 kg. This means that at least 200 mol of ATP (each mole equals 0.5 kg) must be manufactured each day which, in molecular terms, amounts to 12×10^{25} molecules of ATP. Each cell contains about one billion molecules of ATP which are recycled every 20–30 s. During anaerobic metabolism, ATP production falls by more than 90 % and from the above simplified overview, it is patently obvious why such a metabolic state is catastrophic.

The initial priority is to prevent early death from the physiological mayhem of anaerobic metabolism by appropriate resuscitation and surgical intervention, with the secondary goal of preventing late deaths from multiple organ dysfunction (MOD). Interventions undertaken within the first few hours impact heavily on the incidence of MOD, and rapid decisions need to be made, sometimes in the presence of limited information. At every decision point the risk of a particular course of action needs to be weighed against the benefits; acute benefit outweighs later risk. For example, although the use of intravenous contrast during computerized scanning carries the risk of renal damage, it is of enormous benefit in identifying injuries and planning management.

2.1 Converting Anaerobic to Aerobic Metabolism

Although the lethal triad of hypothermia, acidosis, and coagulopathy is a well-accepted consequence of severe hemorrhage [2] and inadequate DO_2, this is a later phase and the forerunners of this have been recognized as hypoxia, hypoperfusion, and hypothermia, the "triple H syndrome" [3]. All three parameters induce a lactic acidosis, have an independent association with mortality, and their correction must be the main aim of resuscitation.

2.1.1 *Hypoxia*

Hypoxia is not synonymous with an abnormal PaO_2 or SaO_2 on blood gas analysis and encompasses the inevitable oxygen debt and accumulation of lactic acid from anaerobic metabolism. The aims of resuscitation are to prevent further accumulation of oxygen debt and institute rapid repayment [4]. Of prime importance is the realization that despite normalizing DO_2, an oxygen debt must still be repaid as indicated by a persistently elevated lactate or base deficit.

Despite an acceptable level of arterial oxygen saturation, endotracheal intubation and mechanical ventilation should be employed liberally in patients with a lactic acidosis. The lungs are the main buffering mechanism by which humans compensate for an acute metabolic acidosis, renal compensation being slower and later, and removing the work of breathing may help substantially. The drug for induction and intubation must be carefully selected in order to avoid further cardiovascular instability, and ketamine and etomidate are the agents of choice despite the reported association of adrenal insufficiency with the latter [5]. This is a late and only potential risk, whereas the effects of hypotension are definite and acute.

Recently the concept of protective lung ventilation (PLV) has been advocated for the critically ill and injured [6], but this is not universally applicable in major trauma, especially during the acute phase. An adequate minute volume is required to buffer a metabolic acidosis; to avoid rises in intracranial pressure following TBI, hypercarbia must be prevented and tidal volumes may need to be higher than those proposed for PLV; and in patients with blunt thoracic trauma and a pulmonary contusion, a substantial proportion of damaged lung may be recruited by initially using higher tidal volumes between 8 and 10 ml/kg. Once recruited the tidal volume may be reduced as necessary, and lung volume maintained with positive end expiratory pressure (PEEP).

2.1.2 Hypoperfusion

Major hemorrhage results in intravascular volume depletion and a significant drop in cardiac output and DO_2. Short periods of hypotension although causing cellular apoptosis result in complete recovery of ATP production, whereas protracted shock episodes cause cell necrosis and irreversible organ damage [7]. The conventional approach has been to restore intravascular volume with clear fluids, either crystalloid or colloid, and augment DO_2 later with blood transfusion. Although restoring intravascular volume and perfusion, clear fluids do not carry oxygen, and a proactive rather than reactive philosophy has recently been adopted with the early use of blood and blood products and limitation of clear resuscitation fluids. To this end a massive transfusion protocol must be established [8] whereby the necessary products are released urgently and as required with the aim of achieving a set ratio of packed red blood cells (PRBCs) to plasma and platelets. This has the desired effect of rapidly optimizing DO_2 and counteracting the effect of the acute coagulopathy of trauma. Experience from military conflicts suggested initially that PRBCs, plasma, and platelets should be administered in a 1:1:1 ratio [9], but evidence from the civilian environment indicates that a less aggressive plasma volume is superior with a PRBC to plasma ratio of 2:1 being preferred, thereby minimizing complications without affecting survival [10].

There is no role for supranormal DO_2, and the use of permissive hypotension is only applicable in the setting of uncontrolled hemorrhage where theater is immediately available. Sustained hypoperfusion results in irreversible organ ischemia and a physiological point of no return.

Consideration should also be given to the early use of vasopressors before full restoration of intravascular volume. This has the effect of constricting nonessential vascular beds and augmenting perfusion to vital organs. Although lactate may rise using this approach, it is not associated with a lactic acidosis but reflects increased glucose metabolism and aerobic lactate formation. Once intravascular volume has been optimized, the vasopressor may be reduced or withdrawn.

The end points of resuscitation are a hemoglobin of 10 g/dl, a platelet count of >50,000, and a near-normal clotting profile. The current evidence recommending a hemoglobin level of between 7 and 9 g/dl in the critically ill [11] pertains only to the later phase of management and is not applicable as an end point in the acute setting. With regard to assessment of coagulation, thromboelastography is far superior to the standard laboratory tests and this equipment should be available as point-of-care testing in the resuscitation area [12]. Lactate and base deficit should be monitored frequently to confirm the reversal of anaerobic metabolism.

The majority of trauma patients respond to these interventions, but on occasion there may be a transient or minimal effect on cardiovascular dynamics. The assumption must be made that hemorrhage is ongoing and the source must be identified; surgical control of hemorrhage is part and parcel of restoring perfusion. The most likely source of concealed hemorrhage is the abdomen or pelvis, and focused abdominal assessment by sonar (FAST) is an essential component during this phase; transporting a hemodynamically unstable patient for computerized scanning must be avoided.

2.1.3 Hypothermia

A reduction in core temperature following major injury is classified as secondary hypothermia which must be distinguished from primary hypothermia where heat production is normal but temperature falls as a result of a cold environment [13]. In secondary hypothermia, heat production is reduced due to a fall in VO_2 which is the main mechanism of heat generation. Following trauma a reduction in core temperature below 35 °C has an independent association with mortality and is universally fatal below 32°. The major detrimental effects of a reduction in core temperature are on coagulation and cardiac function. At a temperature of 35°, clotting times are reduced by more than 50 % and at 33° by more than 80 %. Platelet function is also markedly deranged. Every attempt must be made to avoid this sinister situation, and unlike primary hypothermia, rewarming must be as rapid as possible in patients who are suffering from secondary hypothermia. Foil blankets are completely ineffectual, and peripheral rewarming devices such as convectional air blankets are inefficient for a number of reasons. The inevitable vasoconstriction of hypovolemia prevents heat from being taken up by the peripheral superficial vasculature because skin perfusion may decrease by over 90 % of normal, and according to the second law of thermodynamics, until the peripheral temperature exceeds the core, no heat will be transferred. Their use is mainly to prevent further heat loss. Although all inhaled gases must be warmed and humidified, this is more prophylactic than therapeutic. Core rewarming is the sole effective method and all intravenous fluids must be heated to 40 °C via a dedicated warming device. Placing fluids or blood in buckets of warm water is not recommended. Lavage of the pleural cavity, stomach, or urinary bladder may also be considered although until any injury has been excluded this may be problematic. Continuous arteriovenous rewarming is the most effective method but presents many practical problems in the hemodynamically unstable patient.

2.2   Identification of Injuries and Organ Protection

Once resuscitation is complete, if the physiological state of the patient allows, all injuries need to be identified. For blunt polytrauma computerized scanning with angiography is the gold standard [14], delineates skeletal, soft tissue, and vascular trauma, and allows organ injury severity grading which is essential for planning surgical intervention.

Embarking on prolonged and unnecessary surgery may worsen organ function substantially, and only life- or limb-threatening injuries should be addressed acutely. Competing surgical interests are common in the patient with multiple injuries, the most frequent challenging triad being an intracranial mass lesion, intra-abdominal or pelvic hemorrhage, and peripheral vascular trauma with a threatened limb. In the ideal world, surgery may be undertaken simultaneously if enough personnel are available, but if not, the philosophy must be life over limb. In this scenario, even if repair of a vascular injury to a limb is feasible, if it had occurred in isolation, prolonged surgery may threaten survival and a decision needs to be taken for temporary shunting or primary limb ablation.

Although definitive fracture fixation and the concept of early total care have been reported to decrease organ dysfunction [15], if undertaken too early, the incidence of MOD actually increases [16]. An elevated lactate, even in the presence of normal hemodynamic monitoring, indicates subclinical hypoperfusion and although DO_2 may be normal, an oxygen debt still exists. Definitive fracture management performed at this time is detrimental and should be delayed until lactate has normalized. When non-orthopedic acute surgery is deemed necessary, if fractures coexist, external fixation is the method of choice.

Following any essential surgery, the next phase is to protect body systems from further insult. This involves neuroprotective, lung protective, and renal protective strategies, complemented by global measures to maintain organ function which will be considered in specific chapters. Although a complete appraisal of all injuries is assumed to have been completed by the primary and secondary surveys, a tertiary survey must always be undertaken. Unidentified injuries incur major morbidity and mortality [17], and failure to make the expected recovery or an unexplained deterioration in organ function should raise the suspicion of missed injuries.

The management of the patient with multiple injuries is challenging, demanding, and requires a team approach with input from many disciplines. A trauma surgeon with experience in intensive care must lead the process of decision making, and at each critical point the risk:benefit ratio of any proposed intervention must be carefully assessed.

References

1. Stewart RM, Myers JG, Dent DL et al (2003) Seven hundred fifty-three consecutive deaths in a level I trauma center: the argument for injury prevention. J Trauma 54:66–70
2. Raymer JM, Flynn LM, Martin RF (2012) Massive transfusion of blood in the surgical patient. Surg Clin North Am 92:221–234
3. Muckart DJJ, Bhagwanjee S, Gouws E (1997) Validation of an outcome prediction model for critically ill trauma patients without head injury. J Trauma 43:934–938
4. Barbee RW, Reynolds PS, Ward KR (2010) Assessing shock resuscitation strategies by oxygen debt replacement. Shock 33:113–122

5. Cotton BA, Guillamondegui OD, Flemming SB et al (2008) Increased risk of adrenal insufficiency following etomidate exposure in critically injured patients. Arch Surg 143:62–67

6. The acute respiratory distress syndrome network (2000) Ventilation with lower tidal volumes as compared with traditional tidal volumes for acute lung injury and the acute respiratory distress syndrome. N Engl J Med 342(18):1301–1308

7. Paxian M, Bauer I, Rensing H et al (2003) Recovery of hepatocellular ATP and "pericentral apoptosis" after haemorrhage and resuscitation. FASEB J 17:993–1002

8. Riskin DJ, Tsai TC, Riskin L et al (2009) Massive transfusion protocols: the role of aggressive resuscitation versus product ratio in mortality reduction. J Am Coll Surg 209:198–205

9. Borgman MA, Spinella PC, Perkins JG et al (2007) The ratio of blood products transfused affects mortality in patients receiving massive transfusions at a combat support hospital. J Trauma 63(4):805–813

10. Kashuk JL, Moore EE, Johnson JL et al (2008) Postinjury life threatening coagulopathy: is 1:1 fresh frozen plasma:packed red blood cells the answer? J Trauma 65:261–271

11. McIntyre L, Hebert PC, Wells G et al (2004) Is a restrictive transfusion strategy safe for resuscitated and critically ill trauma patients? J Trauma 57:563–568

12. Kashuk JL, Moore EE (2009) The emerging role of rapid thromboelastography in trauma care. J Trauma 67:417–418

13. Gentilello LM, Pierson DJ (2001) Trauma critical care. Am J Respir Crit Care Med 163:604–607

14. Huber-Wagner S, Lefering R, Qvick LM et al (2009) Effect of whole-body CT during trauma resuscitation on survival: a retrospective, multicentre study. Lancet 373:1455–1461

15. Harwood PJ, Giannoudis PV, van Griensven M et al (2005) Alterations in the systemic inflammatory response after early total care and damage control procedures for femoral shaft fracture in severely injured patients. J Trauma 58:446–452

16. Crowl AC, Young JS, Kahler DM et al (2000) Occult hypoperfusion is associated with increased morbidity in patients undergoing early fracture fixation. J Trauma 48:260–267

17. Muckart DJJ, Thomson SR (1991) Undetected injuries: a preventable cause of increased morbidity and mortality. Am J Surg 162:457–460

Chapter 3
Damage Control Resuscitation

Juan Carlos Duchesne, Bruno Monteiro Pereira, and Gustavo Pereira Fraga

3.1 Introduction

Despite the word "war" refer to a bad feeling, it is undeniable that military conflicts have always driven innovation and technical advances in medicine and surgery. Accepted concepts of trauma resuscitation and surgery have been challenged in the recent wars, and novel approaches have been developed to

J.C. Duchesne, MD, FACS, FCCP, FCCM (✉)
Department of Surgery,
Tulane University,
North Oaks Shock/Trauma Center,
Hammond, LA 70112-2699, USA
e-mail: jduchesn@tulane.edu

B.M. Pereira, MD, MSc, FCCM • G.P. Fraga, MD, PhD, FACS
Division of Trauma Surgery, Department of Surgery,
School of Medical Sciences, University of Campinas,
R. Alexander Fleming, 181 Cidade Univ. Prof. Zeferino Vaz Barao
Geraldo, Campinas, SP 13.083-970, Brazil
e-mail: drbrunomonteiro@hotmail.com; fragagp2008@gmail.com

S. Di Saverio et al. (eds.), *Trauma Surgery*,
DOI 10.1007/978-88-470-5403-5_3, © Springer-Verlag Italia 2014

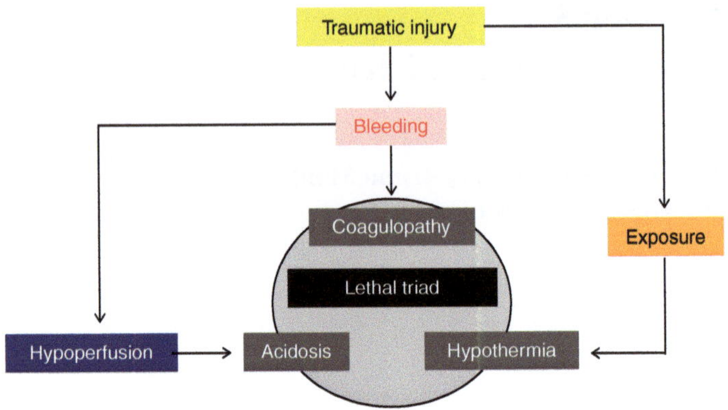

Fig. 3.1 The lethal triad flowchart

address the current complexity and severity of not only military trauma but also civilian conflicts.

Damage control resuscitation (DCR) has become a topic of increasing relevance and popularity over the past several years. Hemorrhage secondary to trauma accounts for 40 % of trauma fatalities and comprises the leading cause of preventable death in trauma [1]. Research in military and civilian populations regarding DCR has focused on ways to improve survival in patients with severe hemorrhage. It should be mentioned that the majority of trauma patients do not require DCR and that its techniques should be reserved for those who are the most severely injured [2]. For these patients the rapid and effective use of techniques to control bleeding and correction of this hemostatic derangement coined as acute coagulopathy of trauma shock (ACoTS) is essential. The perpetuating combination of acute coagulopathy, hypothermia, and acidosis seen in exsanguinating trauma patients is a well-recognized term known as lethal triad (Fig. 3.1). In a practical standpoint, the vicious cycle of acidosis/hypothermia/coagulopathy must be aimed as potential lethal cycle and corrected immediately.

DCR combines two seemingly diverse strategies—permissive hypotension and hemostatic resuscitation—with damage control surgery, integrating these three procedures in one dynamic process. Therefore, DCR is designed to proceed hand in hand with damage control surgery. The sequential strategy of operation followed by resuscitation has been replaced by an integrated approach so that resuscitation and surgery are undertaken simultaneously, with close communication and cooperation between surgeon and anesthetist [2–5].

3.2   Permissive Hypotension

The recognition that fluid resuscitation might interfere with hemostatic mechanisms, ultimately exacerbating blood and coagulation factors loss, led to a reevaluation of the former accepted concept that normal circulatory function is restored by aggressive crystalloids volume. The crystalloid fluid used in initial resuscitative efforts does not contain any clotting factors or erythrocytes. Its use may result in a dilution of clotting factors or role blood and therefore poorer control of bleeding and impaired oxygen transport to tissues causing further ischemic damage. Additionally, crystalloids have an acidic pH, and the administration of large quantities of isotonic or slightly hypertonic crystalloid solutions such as 0.9 % normal saline or lactated Ringer's could cause or aggravate metabolic acidosis, another component of the "lethal triad" leading to a decrease in myocardial function and cell apoptosis [6–9].

Permissive hypotension, also known as hypotensive resuscitation, is a strategy of restricting crystalloids administration until the bleeding is controlled, while accepting a limited period of suboptimum end-organ perfusion.

3.2.1 *Rationale*

Following injury the otherwise healthy individual has a natural ability to clot off bleeding. The higher the vessel pressure, the harder it is for the bleeding to stop, since the fluid essentially "pushes" the clot out and consequently the bleeding resumes. In another words, it is reasonable to think that hypotension facilitates coagulation. Attempts to normalize blood pressure in case of uncontrolled bleeding as in victims of penetrating trauma may result in increased blood loss and worsen outcomes [10]. Another issue with aggressive fluid resuscitation is the potential for hypothermia if fluids that are stored at room temperature are used. If these fluids are not warmed prior to infusion, this can result in a significant drop in core body temperature. As exposed in Fig. 3.1, hypothermia is associated with many problems including bleeding disorder, organ failure, and hypotension and is one of the three components in the "lethal triad," condition that must be feared and soon corrected by all trauma specialists [5–8].

It is important to remember that permissive hypotension is a temporizing measure to improve outcomes until the source of bleeding is controlled. There are consequences associated with prolonged permissive hypotension (>90 min) that must be taken into account. Prolonged permissive hypotension can lead to aggravated post-injury coagulopathy, ischemic damage secondary to poor tissue perfusion including the brain, mitochondrial dysfunction, and lactic acidosis. Permissive hypotension is currently contraindicated in the presence of traumatic brain injury suspicion.

No published evidence exists to support the strategy of permissive or controlled hypotension, although its usefulness has not been entirely ruled out either. Few would argue against replacing lost intravascular volume in patients with controlled or self-limiting hemorrhage. In patients with uncontrolled hemorrhage, particularly in the context of penetrating torso trauma, a strategy of permissive hypotension, together with expert resuscitation and rapid control of hemorrhage, might be more appropriate. It is conceivable that permissive hypotension is more applicable to the management of penetrating trauma, which is often characterized by the presence of major vascular injuries, than to blunt injuries.

Despite the lack of evidence, guideline recommendations for clinical practice point towards judicious administration of intravenous fluids. In recognition of the unique challenges posed by combat casualties, permissive hypotension has been incorporated into military medical doctrine and used widely during the recent war conflicts [4].

3.3 Hemostatic Resuscitation

Hemostatic resuscitation has also recently become a popular form of transfusion therapy. The concept of giving fractionated blood in an attempt to closely approximate whole blood makes a lot of sense. In this context, hemostatic resuscitation provides transfusions with plasma and platelets in addition to red blood cells in an immediate and sustained manner as part of the transfusion protocol for massively bleeding patients. Rapid and proactive treatment of the coagulopathy associated with major injury is now recognized as central to improve outcome. Although early and effective reversal of coagulopathy is documented, the most effective means of preventing coagulopathy of massive transfusion remains debated and randomized controlled studies are lacking [11–14].

With all this said, became clear that the high prevalence and profound impact of coagulopathy mandates timely treatment of trauma patients. Strategies to proactive action in the emergency room and operating room may include administration of packed red blood cells, fresh frozen plasma, and platelets; use of recombinant factor VIIa, cryoprecipitate, and tranexamic acid; and calcium replacement.

Commonly available diagnostic tests—such as prothrombin time and activated partial thromboplastin time—are inappropriate for guiding treatment in trauma patients owing to their poor sensitivity and the delay in obtaining results, so the decision to initiate clotting factor replacement is a clinical one.

3.3.1 Massive Transfusion Protocol

Massive bleeding patients demand a massive transfusion protocol (MTP). The traditional definition of massive transfusion is 20 units red blood cells (RBCs) in 24 h, which corresponds to approximately 1 blood volume in a 70 kg patient. A commonly used definition in the trauma literature is >10 units RBCs in 24 h. Both of these definitions are reasonable for publications, but are not practical in an ongoing resuscitation. Other definitions are loss of 0.5 blood volume within 3 h, use of 50 units of blood components in 24 h, and use of 6 units RBCs in 12 h. From a practical standpoint, requirement for >4 RBC units in 1 h with ongoing need for transfusion or blood loss >150 ml/min with hemodynamic instability and need for transfusion are reasonable definitions in the setting of a MTP situation.

Once MTP is initiated, the target is to achieve a close ratio resuscitation with 1:1:1 of fresh frozen plasma (FFP), platelets (Plts), and packed red blood cells (PRBCs). The rationale behind early and sustained administration of FFP involves the replacement of fibrinogen and clotting factors [15]. In mathematical studies, Hirshberg et al. noted that resuscitation with more than 5 units of PRBCs will lead to a dilutional coagulopathy and that the ideal manner to correct for this coagulopathy would be to add FFP to PRBC in a 2:3 FFP:PRBC ratio [16]. Another study by Ho et al. noted that once excessive deficiency of factors has developed, 1–1.5 units of FFP must be given for every unit of PRBCs transfused [17].

It should be emphasized FFP replacement alone does not address the coagulopathy seen in trauma patients with severe hemorrhage. A quantitative and qualitative platelet dysfunction has been shown to play a role as well in the mechanism of coagulation [18]. Although not as extensively as FFP, platelet replacement as a part of transfusion protocols has been studied to determine the most effective ratio of platelets to PRBC. Hirshberg et al. suggest a ratio of platelet:PRBC of 8:10 is effective in preventing dilution of platelets below the hemostatic threshold [16]. It should be noted, however, that both studies were theoretical models and did not take into account factors such as hypothermia, acidosis, thrombocytopenia, or ACoTS. These mathematical models for FFP and platelets set forth by Hirschberg and Ho have helped modify ratios used for MTPs throughout the world [13, 19].

Approximately 3–5 % of civilian adult trauma patients receive massive transfusion. Early identification of patients requiring MTP has been evaluated by assigning a value of 0 or 1 to the following four parameters: penetrating mechanism, positive FAST for fluid (focused assessment sonography in trauma), arrival blood pressure <90 mmHg, and arrival pulse >120 bpm. A score of 2 or more is considered positive [20–23]. The score is 75 % sensitive and 85 % specific. FAST examination identifies whether there is free fluid within the peritoneum, which could indicate organ rupture and internal bleeding. Patients receiving uncross-matched red cells in the emergency department are three times more likely to receive massive transfusion.

3.3.2 Recombinant Factor VIIa

Recombinant factor VIIa use in trauma emerged because of the additional necessity of correcting ACoTS. Researches suggested that a pharmacological adjunct would be useful to treatment of ACoTS and this could play an important outcome role.

Recombinant activated factor VII (rFVIIa) is a hemostatic agent originally developed to treat hemophilia, FVII deficiency, and Glanzmann thrombasthenia patients refractory to platelet transfusion. The activation of platelets at the site of injury is the reason for a localized action of rFVIIa, as it causes clotting at the site of bleeding. The dose ranges from 60 to 200 g/kg; however, prospective randomized controlled clinical trials using different doses of rFVIIa are needed to explore the potential efficacy of lower doses in traumatic coagulopathy to reduce cost and adverse effects, such as thromboembolic complications [24]. The efficacy and safety of rFVIIa as an adjunct therapy for bleeding control in patients with severe blunt and penetrating trauma were evaluated in a parallel randomized, placebo-controlled, double-blind clinical trial [25]. The authors compared three doses of rFVIIa (doses of 200, 100, and 100 µg/kg) with three doses of placebo in addition to standard treatment in patients who received 6 units of RBCs within a 4-h period. In blunt trauma (143 patients), RBC transfusion was significantly reduced with rFVIIa compared to placebo, and the need for massive transfusion (defined as 20 units of RBCs) was reduced (14 % vs. 33 %, respectively). In penetrating trauma (134 patients), there was no reduction in mortality and complications or reduction of PRBCs transfused in patients receiving rFVIIa. Adverse effects, including thromboembolic events (a total of 12, six in each group), were distributed equally between the groups. The authors concluded that rFVIIa is safe within the investigated dose and may be a promising adjunct to existing therapy in trauma [25]. The effects of liberally administering rFVIIa in hemorrhaging trauma patients are unknown because its procoagulant effect must be balanced against a real risk of thromboembolic events. At present, the use of rFVIIa in correcting coagulopathy from trauma is off-label and has not been approved by the Food and Drug Administration [26].

3.3.3 Fibrinogen and Cryoprecipitate

Fibrinogen deficiency develops earlier than deficiency of other clotting factors. Fibrinogen is, therefore, an obvious target for replacement with either cryoprecipitate—which contains fibrinogen, factor VIII, factor XIII, and von Willebrand factor—or fibrinogen concentrate. Updated guidelines recommend giving either product if plasma fibrinogen levels fall below 1.0 g/l. Concerns about patient exposure to a large number of donors and the associated risk of blood borne virus transmission limit the use of cryoprecipitate to situations where conventional treatment has failed [5, 27].

3.3.4 Tranexamic Acid

Clot breakdown (fibrinolysis) is a normal response to surgery and trauma in order to maintain vascular patency and can become exaggerated (hyperfibrinolysis) in some cases. The anti-fibrinolytic drug tranexamic acid (TXA), a lysine analogue, interferes with the binding of plasminogen to fibrin, which is necessary for plasmin activation. Fibrinolysis consists of acti-vated plamin cleaving fibrin. Antifibrinolytic drugs can prevent clot breakdown and thus reduce blood loss in trauma [28, 29]. TXA has recently been shown to reduce deaths in a large popu-lation of trauma patients. In 2011, the CRASH-2 investigators published an exploratory analysis of the previous trial that spe-cifically evaluated the effect of tranexamic acid on death due to bleeding subdivided by time from treatment to injury. The results showed that earlier treatment with tranexamic acid is more effective in reducing the risk of death due to bleeding. Patients that received tranexamic acid within 1 h of injury had a death rate due to bleeding of 5.3 % versus 7.7 % for placebo (RR 0.79, CI 0.64–0.97; $p < 0.0001$). Similarly, patients that received treatment between 1 and 3 h from injury also had a significantly lower risk of death due to bleeding. However, patients receiving tranexamic acid >3 h from injury had a significantly increased risk of death compared to placebo, 4.4 % versus 3.1 %, respectively (RR 1.44, CI 1.12–1.84; $p=0.004$) [28].

Current recommendations for the use of TXA are the following [29]:

1. Tranexamic acid should be routinely used in trauma patients with evidence of bleeding.
2. Tranexamic acid should be included in transfusion protocols for trauma.
3. Tranexamic acid should be given within 3 h of injury.
4. Administer 1 g of TXA intravenously (bolus over 10 min) followed by the infusion of 1 g over 8 h.

3.3.5 Calcium Administration

Ionized hypocalcaemia is common in critically ill patients and is associated with increased mortality. Calcium is an important cofactor to many components of the coagulation cascade. Citrate, used as an anticoagulant in many blood components, chelates calcium and exacerbates hypocalcaemia. The dose–response effect of hypocalcaemia on coagulation is difficult to measure. A recent nonsystematic review, however, extrapolated that ionized calcium concentrations of less than 0.6–0.7 mmol/l could lead to coagulation defects and recommended maintaining a concentration of at least 0.9 mmol/l [5, 14].

3.3.6 Aged Packed Red Cells

The transfusion of red cells with a high storage age has been associated with increased rates of infective complications and multiple organ failure. Although the shelf life of packed red cell units is around 6 weeks, adverse effects of administration—which are thought to be mediated by passenger leukocytes—have been shown with units at a storage age of about 2 weeks. When blood is stored, the level of antioxidants decreases, resulting in oxidative damage that converts hemoglobin to methemoglobin, which cannot bind to oxygen. If blood is stored for more than 7 days, it loses 2,3-DPG. Without 2,3-DPG, the hemoglobin-oxygen dissociation curve shifts to the left and less oxygen moves into the tissues. Storage also promotes hemolysis and acidosis. Researchers have found that transfused blood is an independent predictor of multisystem organ failure and death [14, 19].

A recent large retrospective cohort study of trauma patients showed that transfusion of red cells stored for longer than 2 weeks was associated with significantly increased odds of death. This finding was observed despite leukoreduction but was apparent only among patients who received at least 6 units of packed cells. Recently donated red cells are, therefore, preferable for trauma patients requiring massive transfusion, although such a practice has obvious logistical and resource implications.

3.4 Damage Control Surgery

The concept of damage control surgery arose from the realization that the massively traumatized patient lacked the physiological reserve to survive the rigors of complex and prolonged definitive or reconstructive surgery. It is now an accepted part of the trauma surgeon's armamentarium and viewed as a component of damage control resuscitation. The aim of damage control surgery is to stop hemorrhage and minimize contamination. Temporary clamping, packing, shunting, or ligation controls hemorrhage, and hollow viscus injuries are either closed or resected without anastomosis. On completion of the procedure, the abdomen is temporarily closed using an improvised or commercially available topical negative pressure dressing, which saves time, helps to minimize the risk of intra-abdominal hypertension, and facilitates observation of the volume and nature of drainage from the abdomen. Planned reoperation to restore anatomy and achieve definitive repair is carried out on return to normal physiology. Damage control surgery is associated with potential morbidity, should be employed judiciously, and should not be practiced in isolation [2, 6, 30].

3.5 Evidence-Based Current Recommendations

3.5.1 Level I Recommendations

An FFP to PRBC ratio of 1:1 is associated with less transfusions. Sufficient evidence does exist for showing that transfusion with FFP will decrease the number of transfusions needed. It should be noted that there are no randomized, prospective, class I trials. Conducting such trials in the future will be essential to continuing to understand the ideal manner to transfuse during trauma.

Class I evidence supports use of antifibrinolytics in massive transfusion. The recently completed CRASH-2 trials demonstrate improved all-cause mortality as well as mortality due to hemorrhage. Further class I, II, and III studies should be performed to further support these findings.

3.5.2 Level II Recommendations

A MTP will improve outcomes for trauma resuscitations. There are many logistical challenges associated with this strategy. Many civilian institutions, even level I trauma centers, have yet to adopt a MTP. However, simple ratios such as 1:1 FFP:PRBC have the benefit of ease of use, and the relatively higher plasma doses appear to be associated with improved outcome. Such a standard protocol can foster multicenter research on resuscitation and hemorrhage control.

High FFP:PRBC is supported by class II and class III evidence and should be considered in the treatment of massively transfused coagulopathic trauma patients. Class II and class III data demonstrates the potential for severe complications such as ARDS/acute lung injury, increased hospital and ICU LOS, and increased ventilator time; however, most studies demonstrate improved mortality, suggesting an overall improvement in the use of these therapies.

3.5.3 Level III Recommendations

Increased FFP to PRBC ratio leads to improved outcomes in massive transfusion with the potential for severe complication. MTP implementation and adherence yields improved results with decreases in mortality and complication rates.

The use of high ratio platelets:PRBC is supported by some class II studies and several class III studies. Increased platelets:PRBC has become an integral part of DCR in recent years.

Several class III studies demonstrate mortality improvement with the use of fibrinogen concentrate. The use of fibrinogen in trauma-induced coagulopathy and DCR should be studied further in class I and class II trials.

Increased FFP to PRBC ratio administered early leads to improved outcomes in massive hemorrhage. This benefit is believed to be extended to patients undergoing transfusion with increased FFP:PRBC ratios due to lower transfusion requirements, less risk of complications secondary to the transfusions, and better ability to compensate for the coagulopathy of trauma. Although there is not yet a consensus regarding mortality reduction from increased FFP:PRBC ratios, there does appear to be a trend towards decreased mortality. Likely optimized protocol guidelines will contribute to standardizing variations among current practices.

References

1. Sauaia A, Moore FA, Moore EE, Moser KS, Brennan R, Read RA et al (1995) Epidemiology of trauma deaths: a reassessment. J Trauma 38(2):185–193
2. Duchesne JC, McSwain NE Jr, Cotton BA, Hunt JP, Dellavolpe J, Lafaro K et al (2010) Damage control resuscitation: the new face of damage control. J Trauma 69(4):976–990
3. Duchesne JC, Holcomb JB (2009) Damage control resuscitation: addressing trauma-induced coagulopathy. Br J Hosp Med (Lond) 70(1):22–25
4. Tarmey NT, Woolley T, Jansen JO, Doran CM, Easby D, Wood PR et al (2012) Evolution of coagulopathy monitoring in military damage-control resuscitation. J Trauma 73(6 Suppl 5):S417–S422
5. Jansen JO, Thomas R, Loudon MA, Brooks A (2009) Damage control resuscitation for patients with major trauma. BMJ 338:b1778
6. Duchesne JC, Barbeau JM, Islam TM, Wahl G, Greiffenstein P, McSwain NE Jr (2011) Damage control resuscitation: from emergency department to the operating room. Am Surg 77(2):201–206
7. Duchesne JC, Guidry C, Hoffman JR, Park TS, Bock J, Lawson S et al (2012) Low-volume resuscitation for severe intraoperative hemorrhage: a step in the right direction. Am Surg 78(9):936–941

8. Duke MD, Guidry C, Guice J, Stuke L, Marr AB, Hunt JP et al (2012) Restrictive fluid resuscitation in combination with damage control resuscitation: time for adaptation. J Trauma 73(3):674–678

9. Spoerke N, Michalek J, Schreiber M, Brasel KJ, Vercruysse G, MacLeod J et al (2011) Crystalloid resuscitation improves survival in trauma patients receiving low ratios of fresh frozen plasma to packed red blood cells. J Trauma 71(2 Suppl 3):S380–S383

10. Mitra B, Cameron PA, Mori A, Fitzgerald M (2012) Acute coagulopathy and early deaths post major trauma. Injury 43(1):22–25

11. Duchesne JC, Hunt JP, Wahl G, Marr AB, Wang YZ, Weintraub SE et al (2008) Review of current blood transfusions strategies in a mature level I trauma center: were we wrong for the last 60 years? J Trauma 65(2):272–278

12. Duchesne JC, Islam TM, Stuke L, Timmer JR, Barbeau JM, Marr AB et al (2009) Hemostatic resuscitation during surgery improves survival in patients with traumatic-induced coagulopathy. J Trauma 67(1): 33–39

13. Gunter OL Jr, Au BK, Isbell JM, Mowery NT, Young PP, Cotton BA (2008) Optimizing outcomes in damage control resuscitation: identifying blood product ratios associated with improved survival. J Trauma 65(3):527–534

14. Holcomb JB, Wade CE, Brasel KJ, Vercruysse G, MacLeod J, Dutton RP et al (2011) Defining present blood component transfusion practices in trauma patients: papers from the Trauma Outcomes Group. J Trauma 71(2 Suppl 3):S315–S317

15. Ketchum L, Hess JR, Hiippala S (2006) Indications for early fresh frozen plasma, cryoprecipitate, and platelet transfusion in trauma. J Trauma 60(6 Suppl):S51–S58

16. Hirshberg A, Dugas M, Banez EI, Scott BG, Wall MJ Jr, Mattox KL (2003) Minimizing dilutional coagulopathy in exsanguinating hemorrhage: a computer simulation. J Trauma 54(3):454–463

17. Ho AM, Dion PW, Cheng CA, Karmakar MK, Cheng G, Peng Z et al (2005) A mathematical model for fresh frozen plasma transfusion strategies during major trauma resuscitation with ongoing hemorrhage. Can J Surg 48(6):470–478

18. Hess JR, Brohi K, Dutton RP, Hauser CJ, Holcomb JB, Kluger Y et al (2008) The coagulopathy of trauma: a review of mechanisms. J Trauma 65(4):748–754

19. Malone DL, Hess JR, Fingerhut A (2006) Massive transfusion practices around the globe and a suggestion for a common massive transfusion protocol. J Trauma 60(6 Suppl):S91–S96

20. Cotton BA, Dossett LA, Haut ER, Shafi S, Nunez TC, Au BK et al (2010) Multicenter validation of a simplified score to predict massive transfusion in trauma. J Trauma 69(Suppl 1):S33–S39
21. Holcomb JB, Zarzabal LA, Michalek JE, Kozar RA, Spinella PC, Perkins JG et al (2011) Increased platelet:RBC ratios are associated with improved survival after massive transfusion. J Trauma 71(2 Suppl 3):S318–S328
22. Nunez TC, Young PP, Holcomb JB, Cotton BA (2010) Creation, implementation, and maturation of a massive transfusion protocol for the exsanguinating trauma patient. J Trauma 68(6):1498–1505
23. Wade CE, del Junco DJ, Holcomb JB, Holcomb JB, Wade CE, Brasel KJ et al (2011) Variations between level I trauma centers in 24-hour mortality in severely injured patients requiring a massive transfusion. J Trauma 71(2 Suppl 3):S389–S393
24. Duchesne JC, Mathew KA, Marr AB, Pinsky MR, Barbeau JM, McSwain NE (2008) Current evidence based guidelines for factor VIIa use in trauma: the good, the bad, and the ugly. Am Surg 74(12): 1159–1165
25. Mitra B, Mori A, Cameron PA, Fitzgerald M, Paul E, Street A (2010) Fresh frozen plasma (FFP) use during massive blood transfusion in trauma resuscitation. Injury 41(1):35–39
26. Fraga GP, Bansal V, Coimbra R (2010) Transfusion of blood products in trauma: an update. J Emerg Med 39(2):253–260
27. Duchesne JC (2011) Lyophilized fibrinogen for hemorrhage after trauma. J Trauma 70(5 Suppl):S50–S52
28. Roberts I, Shakur H, Afolabi A, Brohi K, Coats T, Dewan Y et al (2011) The importance of early treatment with tranexamic acid in bleeding trauma patients: an exploratory analysis of the CRASH-2 randomised controlled trial. Lancet 377(9771):1096–1101
29. Luz L, Sankarankutty A, Passos E, Rizoli S, Fraga GP, Nascimento B Jr (2012) Tranexamic acid for traumatic hemorrhage. Rev Col Bras Cir 39(1):77–80
30. Duchesne JC, Kimonis K, Marr AB, Rennie KV, Wahl G, Wells JE et al (2010) Damage control resuscitation in combination with damage control laparotomy: a survival advantage. J Trauma 69(1):46–52

Chapter 4
Principles and Philosophy
of Damage Control Surgery

Fredric M. Pieracci and Ernest E. Moore

This technique of initial abortion of laparotomy, establishment of intra-abdominal pack tamponade, and then completion of the surgical procedure once coagulation has returned to an acceptable level has proven to be lifesaving in previously non-salvageable situations.

– Harlan Stone, 1983 [1]

The term "damage control" originated within the US Navy and referred to doing the minimum amount necessary with limited resources in the face of a catastrophe to keep a vessel afloat until help arrived. This concept was then applied to trauma surgery in response to advancements in the understanding of hemorrhagic shock. Specifically, the potentiating effects of hypothermia, acidosis, and coagulopathy, referred to as the bloody viscous cycle [2], are now understood to eventuate in exsanguination that cannot be stopped by mechanical surgical interventions. The high mortality associated with the development of the bloody viscous cycle led surgeons to investigate alternatives to lengthy, complicated initial operations in exsanguinating trauma patients. From this experimentation arose the damage control approach, which addresses the problem of nonsurgical coagulopathy by

F.M. Pieracci, MD, MPH (✉) • E.E. Moore, MD
Department of Surgery, Denver Health Medical Center,
777 Bannock Street, MC 0206, Denver, CO 80206, USA
e-mail: fredric.pieracci@dhha.org; ernest.moore@dhha.org

S. Di Saverio et al. (eds.), *Trauma Surgery*,
DOI 10.1007/978-88-470-5403-5_4, © Springer-Verlag Italia 2014

performing an abbreviated initial operation, centered upon rapidly controlling immediately life-threatening injuries, followed by goal-directed resuscitation in the controlled setting of the intensive care unit (ICU), and after temporarily packing and closing body cavities to limit further blood, protein, and heat loss. Only after restoration of metabolic and coagulation integrity does the patient return to the operating room for definitive repair of injuries. Originally described in the setting of abdominal trauma, the damage control approach has now been applied to a variety of body regions, including thoracic, orthopedic, and neurosurgical; many of these specific areas are presented in further detail throughout this text. Most recently, the damage control approach has been extended beyond the realm of trauma into that of emergency general surgery [3]. The success of the damage control approach brought forth new challenges; the management of open, edematous body cavities, particularly the open abdomen, has become a necessary topic of discussion as a direct consequence of survival following damage control surgery. This chapter will review the indications for, technique of, and sequelae of damage control surgery.

4.1 What Is Damage Control Surgery?

Broadly defined, the damage control approach begins with an abbreviated initial surgery in the face of profound hemorrhagic shock, the goal of which is to preserve life. This philosophy is contingent upon an understanding of the negative impact that metabolic failure has on the ability of the trauma patient to tolerate further surgical insults. Specifically, hemorrhage, in conjunction with radiant heat loss from exposed body cavities, and compounded by additional tissue trauma from further dissection, results in acidosis, hypothermia, and coagulopathy. These three basic factors constitute a "bloody viscous cycle," positively feeding back upon one another and eventuating in mortality from exsanguination. Any further operative maneuvers in this setting serve only to exacerbate the cycle, as mechanical bleeding is not the primary source of the problem. Accordingly, the damage control approach involves doing the least amount of operating to save the patient's life and temporarily close body cavities. Surgical hemorrhage is stopped via packing, ligation, or shunting, and gross contamination from the gastrointestinal tract is addressed by rapid over sewing or stapling. Anything more complicated than this, such as vascular anastomosis or bypass grafting, intestinal resection, anastomosis, or enteral feeding access, should not be undertaken during the initial operation. The damage control approach is thus predicated on the somewhat counterintuitive surgical principle of "less is more." Because the temptation in the face of bleeding and shock is to keep operating, adoption of the damage control approach requires both self-control, resisting the urge to expose the unstable trauma patient to additional unhelpful operative insults, and the perspective to address the overall clinical scenario rather than individual injuries. Definitive repair of injuries and fascial closure is forgone for hours to days until after a period of resuscitation in the ICU.

4.2 What Is the History of Damage Control Surgery?

The surgical approach that has recently been termed damage control has existed for over 100 years. Both Pringle [4] and Halstead [5] outlined the utility of packing for management of hepatic trauma in the early twentieth century. However, as surgical techniques improved, packing for control of hepatic hemorrhage fell out of favor and was almost universally abandoned following World War II. One major concern at the time involved infection from retained packs, and surgeons such as Madding emphatically asserted that abdominal packs were to be removed prior to the end of the operation [6]. By the early 1970s, advances in transport of trauma patients increased the number of patients presenting to major trauma centers who were exsanguinating but salvageable. Accordingly, renewed interest in temporary packing in highly select patients arose. Reports of success began to surface in small groups of patients using hepatic packing specifically. In 1976, Lucas and Ledgerwood described a prospective 5-year evaluation of 637 patients treated for severe liver injury [7]. Packs were inserted in only three patients, all of whom survived. At the 1979 meeting of the Southwestern Surgical Congress, our group reported that over 80 % of deaths from liver trauma were due to uncontrollable, nonsurgical hemorrhage, strengthening the concept of post-injury coagulopathy and the merits of abbreviated laparotomy with packing [2]. Calne et al. [8] and Feliciano et al. [9] soon followed with case series of nearly 100 % survival following hepatic packing.

A landmark study in the evolution of the contemporary damage control sequence was performed by Stone et al. in 1983 [1]. Trauma patients who developed a major coagulopathy during laparotomy were managed either by completion of the procedure in detail or by abortion of the procedure, intra-abdominal packing, and return for definitive repair once coagulation status had normalized. Eleven of 17 (64.7 %) patients managed with abbreviated laparotomy survived, whereas only 1 of 14 (7.1 %) patients with definitive repair during the initial procedure lived. From these studies as well as their own experience, Rotondo and Schwab et al. popularized the term "damage control" within the discipline of trauma surgery [10]. Shortly after, Moore detailed the five classic stages in our current damage control sequence [11].

4.3   What Are the Stages of Damage Control Surgery?

Once initiated, the damage control sequence follows specific stages that begin and end at predetermined time points. Transition through stages is triggered by the overall hemodynamic and metabolic states of the patient.

Stage I, Patient Selection for Abbreviated Laparotomy: The initial step in the damage control sequence involves rapid identification of patients who will benefit from this approach. Although the decision to perform damage control surgery is often made intraoperatively, certain risk factors are recognized to increase the likelihood of damage control and thus may be used to anticipate this decision in the preoperative setting and prepare accordingly. These parameters are summarized in Table 4.1. In general, hemodynamic instability with a presumed thoracic, abdominal, pelvic, or extremity vascular injury should initiate preparation for a damage control approach. Patients who survive emergency department thoracotomy and are transported to the operative room are also included in this subset. Patients who require multiple emergency procedures (e.g., craniotomy and laparotomy) should also be considered for damage control.

Table 4.1 Cases in which damage control should be considered preoperatively

High-energy blunt torso trauma
Multiple torso penetrations
Hemodynamic instability
Presenting coagulopathy and/or hypothermia
Major abdominal vascular injury with multiple visceral injuries
Multifocal or multi-cavity exsanguination with visceral injuries
Multiregional injury with competing priorities

When the decision to pursue damage control surgery has been made preoperatively, minimal additional evaluation in the emergency department is necessary prior to transporting the patient to the operating room. Time spent in the emergency room should be limited to establishment of a definitive airway and intravenous access and evaluation for both pneumothorax/massive hemothorax (via physical exam with or without chest radiography) and pericardial hemorrhage (via focused examination of the abdomen for trauma).

When made intraoperatively, the decision to perform damage control surgery is based broadly upon the six variables outlined in Table 4.2. After initial control of major bleeding and gastrointestinal contamination, an overall assessment of the patient's metabolic and coagulation integrity is made by querying the following parameters: (1) hemodynamic status, (2) metabolic status, (3) temperature, (4) coagulation status, and (5) clinical assessment of nonsurgical bleeding. Hypotension from hemorrhagic shock is a clear indication to perform damage control. However, more subtle indicators of shock, such as increasing vasopressor requirements, hypocapnia, and metabolic acidosis, should all be evaluated. This task requires frequent and clear communication with the anesthesiology team. Patient temperature and coagulation status should be monitored frequently. Routine coagulation parameters, such as the activated partial thromboplastin time, prothrombin time, and international normalized ratio, are insensitive in detecting coagulopathy because they measure only the earliest stages of clot formation. Furthermore, results of these tests are typically not available immediately. For these reasons, we prefer point-of-care thromboelastography (TEG) [12]. Finally, the astute clinician will recognize the development of nonsurgical bleeding as evidenced by hemorrhage from raw surfaces, needle holes, and intravenous catheter sites. These findings signify the development of profound coagulopathy and mandate damage control surgery.

Table 4.2 Cases in which damage control should be considered intraoperatively

Indication	Example
Inability to achieve hemostasis secondary to a recalcitrant coagulopathy	Massive transfusion with disseminated intravascular coagulation
Inaccessible major venous injury	Retrohepatic vena caval disruption
Anticipated need for a time-consuming procedure	Pancreaticoduodenectomy
Demand for nonoperative control of extra-abdominal life-threatening injuries	Ruptured pelvic fracture hematoma requiring selective arterial embolization
Inability to approximate the abdominal incision due to extensive splanchnic reperfusion-induced visceral edema	Protracted shock with massive fluid administration
Desire to reassess abdominal contents	Extensive mesenteric venous injury

Although the technical aspects of the abridged laparotomy are dictated by the injury pattern, in general, the initial damage control operation is divided into three sequential steps: (1) control of hemorrhage, (2) control of gastrointestinal contamination, and (3) temporary closure. Hemorrhage may be controlled by a variety of maneuvers, including packing, ligation, and shunting. In general, venous bleeding may be controlled by pressure pack tamponade using laparotomy pads. The packs are then left in place for transport to the ICU and removal at reoperation. By contrast, arterial or portal venous bleeding requires control with suture repair, ligation, or shunting. Under the extreme conditions of damage control, ligation of almost any vessel is compatible with life. If hemorrhage control can only be accomplished by manual pressure (e.g., sponge stick tamponade of an inferior vena cava injury prior to obtaining proximal and distal control), the surgeon should do so in order to allow for crystalloid and blood product resuscitation prior to exposing the patient to further hemorrhage. In extreme circumstances, control of hemorrhage may be possible only by cross-clamping of the abdominal aorta. Patients may be transported to the ICU with the clamp in place, provided that it is moved to an infrarenal location and that the cross-clamp time is monitored carefully, with flow being reestablished intermittently by transient release of the clamp. Control of gastrointestinal perforation is accomplished by rapid closure using either suture or staples. Although this phase of the operation should proceed rapidly, it should not be haphazard. Poorly placed sutures in tenuous areas such as the esophagus or duodenum may lead to catastrophic consequences subsequently provided that the patient survives, and the surgeon should take the extra few seconds to ensure proper suture placement through viable tissue and complete wound closure.

During the initial operation, efforts should be made to minimize both hypothermia and coagulopathy. Techniques to both prevent and reverse hypothermia include increasing the operating room temperature to >30 °C, infusing warmed fluids, covering body areas not in the operative field with warming devices, and using warmed irrigation fluid. Restoration of clotting function should be goal-directed using serial TEG tracings. When this method is not possible, blood component therapy should be replaced with a ratio of RBC/FFP/plts/cryoprecipitate of approximately 10:5:1:1 [13].

Stage II, Reassessment for Hemorrhage Control: An often underemphasized issue in the damage control literature involves the decision of when to transfer the patient from the operating room to the ICU. Although prompt transfer is both rational and cost-effective, premature departure with ongoing mechanical bleeding may lead to an inexorable bloody viscous cycle in the ICU. Finally, there are select cases in which packing may not be necessary and fascial closure is possible once coagulation integrity has been restored.

In cases of ongoing bleeding, a determination that the current amount of hemorrhage is "acceptable" as being nonsurgical must be made. Although this decision may be guided by the development of obvious nonsurgical bleeding (e.g., from intravenous sites), it is the authors' contention that this decision is often made too late and the operation continued unnecessarily. One technique to aid in this determination is temporary (i.e., 20–30 min) abdominal closure with towel clips (Fig. 4.1), followed by reopening and assessment of the amount of residual intra-abdominal hemorrhage. During this time, collective (i.e., surgery, anesthesia, blood bank) efforts are focused on normalizing temperature, acid–base status, and coagulopathy and critically reevaluating patient salvageability. One important exception to this practice is an isolated pelvic fracture with arterial hemorrhage, which warrants immediate angiographic intervention.

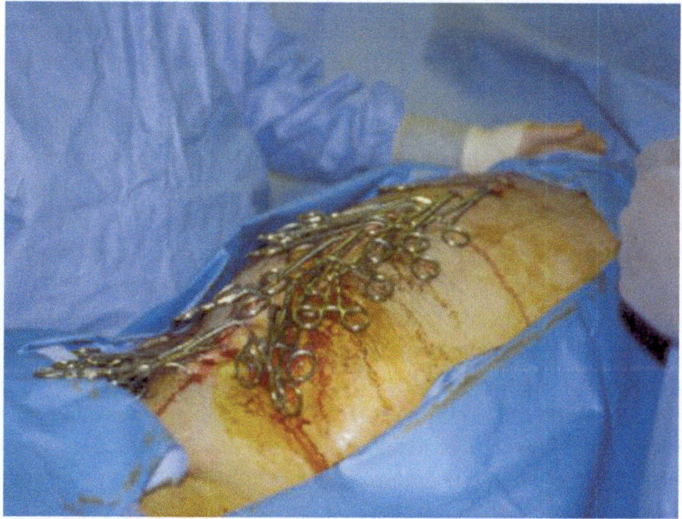

Fig. 4.1 Towel-clipped abdomen

After the brief period of towel clamp closure, the abdomen is examined for residual hemorrhage. Packs, except those successfully tamponading major hepatic venous injuries, are withdrawn sequentially to determine both efficacy and necessity (there are cases, although relatively infrequent, in which the packing can be completely removed and the fascia closed without incident). At this time, a search is undertaken for both residual mechanical bleeding and missed gastrointestinal injuries. In general, if more blood is present in the abdominal cavity than has been transfused during the period of towel clamping, surgical bleeding still exists and should be investigated. By contrast, bleeding from coagulopathy will only worsen if the operation is continued, and in this case, the patient should be closed temporarily and transported to the ICU, at which time damage control stage III begins. Although it is often uncomfortable to stop operating on a patient who is still bleeding, in the setting of profound shock and coagulopathy, this decision is usually lifesaving.

The final step in damage control stage II involves temporary wound closure. In the case of thoracic damage control via a lateral thoracotomy incision, the most rapid and simple technique involves stapled closure of skin only over tube thoracostomy drainage. In the case of a sternotomy, application of an adhesive, translucent dressing over the wound is sufficient. More options exist for laparotomy wound closure, ranging from towel clipping to achieve further tamponade to insertion of a translucent plastic dressing over the abdominal contents, over which drains may be placed and connected to a continuous suction to manage fluid efflux and monitor ongoing hemorrhage (Fig. 4.2). Disadvantages of the towel clip method include an increased likelihood of abdominal compartment syndrome (ACS) and inability to visualize the underlying bowel. Disadvantages of the latter method involve promotion of ongoing hemorrhage from the closed suction drains. None of these techniques has been proven superior to the others, and the overarching principle of rapid, controlled closure should not be overshadowed by the specifics of the dressing.

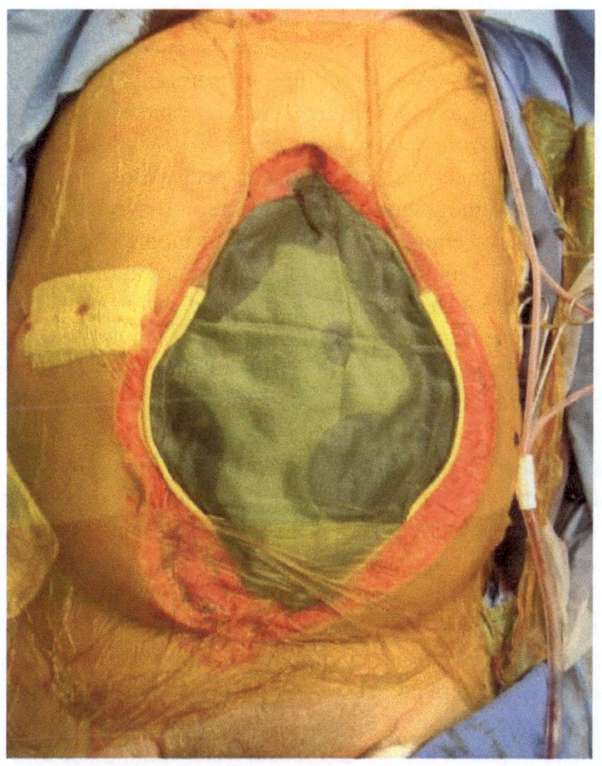

Fig. 4.2 Temporary abdominal closure with green towel, Jackson Pratt drains, and Betadine-impregnated adhesive dressing

Stage III, Physiologic Restoration in the ICU: The patient for whom a damage control approach has been selected usually arrives to the ICU in shock. As such, damage control stage III is centered on resuscitation. Hypothermia and coagulopathy are reversed aggressively. We favor goal-directed restoration of both enzymatic and platelet clotting function using serial TEG tracings. Although the optimal hemoglobin concentration during resuscitation from hemorrhagic shock remains unknown, a concentration of 8–10 g/dL is reasonable, and the decision to transfuse pRBCs should be based primarily upon clinical parameters (e.g., hemodynamic instability) and estimated ongoing blood loss from open wounds and drains. Many endpoints of resuscitation, such as serum lactate concentration, base deficit, and venous hemoglobin oxygen saturation, have been debated and are likely equivalent in terms of monitoring progress. Regardless of which marker is chosen, resuscitation should be guided by serial determinations and stop when normalization has occurred. Furthermore, utilization of multiple markers should be employed, such that the overall clinical picture is given preference over any one laboratory value. This strategy minimizes the possibility of misinterpreting isolated values and either terminating resuscitation prematurely or continuing with unnecessary and potentially deleterious volume expansion. A worsening base deficit in the otherwise resuscitated patient is usually due to a metabolic acidosis from large volume infusion of chloride-rich fluids (e.g., normal saline). Calculation of both the anion gap and serum chloride concentration will aid in this determination; a non-anion gap, hyperchloremic metabolic acidosis is characteristic. A worsening or persistently elevated lactate concentration in the otherwise resuscitated patient may be due to impaired hepatic clearance. Determination of a lactate/pyruvate ratio will elucidate this cause.

During damage control stage III, all organ systems should be supported, and no attempts at either liberation from mechanical ventilation or institution of enteral nutrition should be made until the patient is fully resuscitated. However, once resuscitated, institution of enteral nutrition (provided that the gastrointestinal tract is in continuity) is associated with improved subsequent fascial closure rates, morbidity, and mortality in open abdomen patients without associated intestinal injury and equivalent outcomes in those patients with associated intestinal injury [14]. It is thus the authors' practice to institute enteral nutrition in the resuscitated damage control patient with an open abdomen.

Once the patient is warmed, and both enzymatic and platelet coagulopathy and metabolic derangements have been corrected, consideration is given to progression to damage control stage IV. It is important to recognize that, in contrast to the initial operation of damage control stage I, the reoperation of damage control stage IV is non-emergent. As such, the operation should occur after ensuring availability of blood products, personnel, and equipment. Abundant data now exists documenting the safety of maintaining intracorporeal laparotomy pads, indwelling vascular shunts, and gastrointestinal discontinuity for hours to days. Furthermore, time should be taken during damage control stage III to conduct a thorough evaluation for associated injuries that may have been overlooked heretofore.

Two instances in which consideration should be given to earlier return to the operation room warrant discussion. The first involves concern for ongoing surgical bleeding. Although differentiation from diffuse coagulopathy is often difficult, Morris et al. proposed indications for emergent reoperation during damage control phase III: for blunt trauma, normothermia with a rate of hemorrhage of >2 units pRBC per hour and, for penetrating trauma, either hypothermia with a hemorrhage rate of >15 units pRBC per hour or normothermia with a hemorrhage rate of >2 units pRBC per hour [15]. The second instance in which reoperation should be considered earlier is when the viability of bowel is in question, as is the case following ligation of a major mesenteric vein such as the portal or superior mesenteric. Furthermore, any patient who remains acidotic following correction of temperature, anemia, and coagulation status should be reexplored early with the specific concern of intestinal necrosis.

Stage IV, Return to the Operating Room for Definitive Procedures: At planned reoperation, intra-abdominal packing is removed, definitive vascular and intestinal tract repair is accomplished, a thorough exploration for missed injuries is undertaken, and fascial and skin closure may be performed provided that there is adequate laxity of the anterior abdominal wall tissues, and risk factors for the development of ACS are absent (discussed below). Packing should be removed carefully and after wetting to prevent dislodgement of formed clot. Persistent venous hemorrhage may necessitate repacking and a planned third operation.

Both options and techniques for definitive repair of specific injuries are discussed elsewhere in this text. Once definitive repairs have been achieved, and additional missed injuries have been excluded, a decision regarding fascial closure is made. In certain instances abdominal wall and bowel wall edema is so pronounced that fascial closure is obviously impossible. In the remainder of cases, consideration is given to both the anticipated volume of postoperative fluid resuscitation and the amount of physiologic derangement caused by fascial closure. One useful test involves temporarily re-approximating the fascia with towel clips and monitoring the patient's airway pressure. A steep rise in either peak or mean airway pressures signifies a high likelihood of ACS following fascial closure.

Patients in whom definitive fascial closure is achieved following damage control phase IV must be monitored aggressively for the development of ACS. Intra-abdominal hypertension leading to ACS is a particularly devastating complication of damage control surgery with a high associated morbidity and mortality [16]. The pathophysiology of ACS involves a progressive increase in abdominal pressure due to any combination of diminished abdominal wall compliance, increased intraluminal intestinal contents, increased intraperitoneal fluid, and increased tissue edema. Increases in abdominal pressure eventually become sufficient to impede venous return from both abdominal viscera (resulting in intestinal ischemia) and the inferior vena cava (causing decreased filling pressures and obstructive shock). Both impedance of urinary drainage and respiratory embarrassment secondary to elevated airway pressures are also characteristic. Several risk factors for ACS are recognized; fascial closure during damage control stage IV has been identified repeatedly as a risk factor for the development of ACS. Both large volume fluid resuscitation and attempts to resuscitate to supranormal physiology have also been implicated [17–19].

Physical exam findings, such as elevated airway pressures, oliguria, and tube feeding intolerance, may aid in the diagnosis of abdominal hypertension, but are in and of themselves insensitive [20, 21], mandating measurement of intra-abdominal pressure. Several techniques have been described, including transduction of intragastric, intravesicular, and intraperitoneal pressure. Measurement of the intravesicular pressure is the current reference standard with several noteworthy technical considerations. Measurement should occur at the midaxillary line, at end expiration, in the absence of muscle contractions, and after instilling no more than 25 mL of sterile saline into the urinary bladder [16]. Pressure is expressed as mm Hg. Normal intra-abdominal pressure is <7 mmHg, increases >12 mmHg constitute abdominal hypertension, and a sustained pressure ≥20 mmHg in the presence of organ failure is diagnostic of ACS. Disease severity may also be expressed as the abdominal perfusion pressure, defined as the mean arterial pressure minus the intra-abdominal pressure. An abdominal perfusion pressure <50–60 mmHg is associated with poor outcomes among patients with intra-abdominal hypertension [22].

Medical therapy aimed at reducing abdominal pressure may be attempted for the hemodynamically stable patient in the absence of worsening organ failure. Paralysis, intestinal decompression, and diuresis are all effective means to decrease abdominal pressure. However, sustained or worsening intra-abdominal hypertension after a brief trial of nonoperative maneuvers mandates surgical decompression, as delay in definitive decompression worsens outcomes substantially [22]. Percutaneous catheter decompression may be considered when elevated abdominal pressure is secondary to intraperitoneal fluid (e.g., ascites). Small case series suggest that this technique may be particularly useful among burn patients [23–25]. However, beyond this specific circumstance, surgical decompression via laparotomy remains the definitive treatment for ACS. Failure of improvement following surgical decompression should raise concern for either inadequate decompression or misdiagnosis. When timely and effective surgical decompression is achieved, the abdomen is usually amenable to closure within 7 days.

Stage V, Abdominal Wall Reconstruction: When fascial closure is not possible at the time of damage control phase IV, a variety of methods exist for temporary abdominal dressing, ranging from intravenous solution bags to vacuum-assisted closure devices. General management principles for the open abdomen in the acute setting include wound care, fluid and electrolyte balance, nutritional support, and attempts at sequential closure. Provided an adequate dressing is in place, patients with an open abdomen may be awoken, extubated, and participate in their care and medical decision making. Although evisceration around the abdominal dressing with abrupt increases in intra-abdominal pressure is possible (e.g., coughing fits), this risks is overshadowed by the potential complications of prolonged sedation, paralysis, and mechanical ventilation.

During the immediate postoperative days to weeks, our practice is to perform sequential washouts and partial primary closures approximately every 48 h with the goal of ultimate fascial closure during the index hospitalization. This technique involves sequential primary re-approximation of the midline fascia with interrupted suture bites over a vacuum-assisted closure sponge [26]. Because all damage control patients are markedly total body volume overloaded, aggressive diuresis is helpful to maximize the likelihood of fascial closure, provided that renal and cardiac function will tolerate it. As mentioned previously, enteral nutrition is not contraindicated in the patient with an open abdomen and likely improves outcomes [14]. Using a standardized protocol that incorporates these principles, we are able to achieve fascial closure in nearly all damage control patients during the index hospitalization [26].

The incidence of complications associated with the acutely open abdomen raises sharply after a period of 1–2 weeks [27]. The two most devastating complications are entero-atmospheric fistulae and tertiary peritonitis. The term entero-atmospheric fistula refers to a communication between a hollow viscus and ambient air through the open abdominal incision (as opposed to through the skin in the case of an entero-*cutaneous* fistula). The risk of entero-atmospheric fistula increases linearly with time as a consequence of multiple dressing changes and prolonged exposure and manipulation of the vulnerable, edematous intestinal contents. Entero-atmospheric fistulae are particularly difficult to manage due to the lack of surrounding skin to which dressing appliances may be secured.

Tertiary peritonitis refers to persistent infection of the abdominal cavity despite multiple attempts at source control [28]. At the cellular level, tertiary peritonitis is characterized by failure of host peritoneal defense mechanisms, such that infection is encountered at each reoperation despite prior efforts to eradicate it. Although the peritoneal cavity is initially continuous, adhesions that form over days to weeks partition the space into multiple potential sites of abscess formation, including sub-diaphragmatic, inter-loop, and pelvic. As time elapses, these cavities become increasingly difficult to drain effectively, and the benefit of drainage is rapidly outweighed by the risk of bowel injury from repeated manipulation. As opposed to secondary peritonitis, the microbiology of tertiary peritonitis is characterized by a high prevalence of multidrug-resistant organisms such as enterococci, *Pseudomonas aeruginosa*, and *Candida* spp., making effective antimicrobial therapy challenging.

The best treatment of both entero-atmospheric fistulae and tertiary peritonitis is prevention. Accordingly, if fascial closure of the open abdomen is not possible after 1–2 weeks, we advocate temporarily skin closure over the abdominal contents, either with native skin (provided there is enough laxity) or autologous, split-thickness skin grafting from another site. Although this approach relegates the patient to a planned ventral hernia, the aforementioned complications of the open abdomen are minimized. Definitive fascial closure using more complex techniques, such as component separation and myocutaneous advancement flaps, should not be attempted in the acute setting, especially in the setting of peritonitis. Rather, development of the planes necessary for these operations should be reserved for the elective setting, at which time the risk of recurrence is much lower.

The time period following hospital discharge with a planned ventral hernia represents the final period in the damage control sequence [29]. Techniques for late closure are many and beyond the scope of this chapter. In the majority of cases, a combination of techniques, in conjunction with assistance from a plastic surgeon, can achieve definitive fascial closure with durable results and minimal morbidity.

Damage Control Ground Zero: Several authors have expanded the damage control concept to include the time between initial insult and operation, termed damage control ground zero. This phase highlights the importance of triage, emergency medical services scene time, rewarming in the trauma bay, early injury pattern recognition, and the early decision to initiate the damage control sequence. As mentioned previously, once the decision to initiate damage control has been made, minimal additional time should be spent in the emergency department prior to operation.

4.4 What Has Been the Impact of Damage Control Surgery on Patient Outcomes?

Since the initial description of the damage control technique, many groups have published data detailing improved outcomes using this approach. Although no randomized trials exist, several carefully matched case control series have concluded that mortality is decreased following adoption of damage control, provided that both appropriate indications and triggers for progression through the sequence exist [30, 31]. These improved outcomes are likely multifactorial in etiology, including broadened threshold to initiate damage control, earlier decision to terminate the initial operation, improved ICU resuscitation, and advancements in the techniques for achieving definite abdominal closure.

4.5 Summary

The damage control approach recognizes the notion that prolonged operation in the face of both shock and coagulopathy increases mortality. It is thus predicated on an initial, abbreviated, lifesaving laparotomy, followed by a period of resuscitation in the ICU, and finally by a planned reoperation at which definitive repair is accomplished. Multiple factors contribute to the decision to initiate the damage control sequence and can be broadly grouped into the physiologic variables of hemodynamics, temperature, metabolism of acid, and coagulopathy. A necessary sequelae of the damage control approach is the open abdomen. Although a variety of management options exist, of paramount importance is achieving coverage of intestinal contents so as to minimize the development of fistulae and peritonitis. Adoption of the damage control approach has been associated with markedly improved outcomes for the sickest injured patients and should be part of the armamentarium of all traumatologists.

References

1. Stone HH, Strom PR, Mullins RJ (1983) Management of the major coagulopathy with onset during laparotomy. Ann Surg 197:532–535
2. Kashuk JL, Moore EE, Millikan JS, Moore JB (1982) Major abdominal vascular trauma – a unified approach. J Trauma 22:672–679
3. Stawicki SP, Brooks A, Bilski T, Scaff D, Gupta R, Schwab CW et al (2008) The concept of damage control: extending the paradigm to emergency general surgery. Injury 39:93–101
4. Pringle JH (1908) V. Notes on the arrest of hepatic hemorrhage due to trauma. Ann Surg 48:541–549
5. Halsted WS (1913) V. Partial occlusion of the thoracic and abdominal aortas by bands of fresh aorta and of fascia lata. Ann Surg 58:183–187
6. Madding GF (1955) Injuries of the liver. AMA Arch Surg 70:748–756
7. Lucas CE, Ledgerwood AM (1976) Prospective evaluation of hemostatic techniques for liver injuries. J Trauma 16:442–451
8. Calne RY, McMaster P, Pentlow BD (1979) The treatment of major liver trauma by primary packing with transfer of the patient for definitive treatment. Br J Surg 66:338–339
9. Feliciano DV, Mattox KL, Burch JM, Bitondo CG, Jordan GL Jr (1986) Packing for control of hepatic hemorrhage. J Trauma 26:738–743
10. Rotondo MF, Schwab CW, McGonigal MD, Phillips GR 3rd, Fruchterman TM, Kauder DR et al (1993) 'Damage control': an approach for improved survival in exsanguinating penetrating abdominal injury. J Trauma 35:375–382; discussion 382–383
11. Moore EE, Thomas G (1996) Orr Memorial Lecture. Staged laparotomy for the hypothermia, acidosis, and coagulopathy syndrome. Am J Surg 172:405–410

12. Gonzalez E, Pieracci FM, Moore EE, Kashuk JL (2010) Coagulation abnormalities in the trauma patient: the role of point-of-care thromboelastography. Semin Thromb Hemost 36:723–737
13. Kashuk JL, Moore EE, Johnson JL, Haenel J, Wilson M, Moore JB et al (2008) Postinjury life threatening coagulopathy: is 1:1 fresh frozen plasma:packed red blood cells the answer? J Trauma 65:261–270; discussion 270–271
14. Burlew CC, Moore EE, Cuschieri J, Jurkovich GJ, Codner P, Nirula R et al (2012) Who should we feed? A Western Trauma Association multi-institutional study of enteral nutrition in the open abdomen after injury. J Trauma Acute Care Surg 73(6):1380–1387
15. Morris JA Jr, Eddy VA, Rutherford EJ (1996) The trauma celiotomy: the evolving concepts of damage control. Curr Probl Surg 33:611–700
16. Cheatham ML, Malbrain ML, Kirkpatrick A, Sugrue M, Parr M, De Waele J et al (2007) Results from the International Conference of Experts on Intra-abdominal Hypertension and Abdominal Compartment Syndrome. II. Recommendations. Intensive Care Med 33:951–962
17. Malbrain ML, Chiumello D, Pelosi P, Bihari D, Innes R, Ranieri VM et al (2005) Incidence and prognosis of intraabdominal hypertension in a mixed population of critically ill patients: a multiple-center epidemiological study. Crit Care Med 33:315–322
18. Balogh Z, McKinley BA, Cocanour CS, Kozar RA, Valdivia A, Sailors RM et al (2003) Supranormal trauma resuscitation causes more cases of abdominal compartment syndrome. Arch Surg 138:637–642; discussion 642–643
19. Madigan MC, Kemp CD, Johnson JC, Cotton BA (2008) Secondary abdominal compartment syndrome after severe extremity injury: are early, aggressive fluid resuscitation strategies to blame? J Trauma 64:280–285
20. Kirkpatrick AW, Brenneman FD, McLean RF, Rapanos T, Boulanger BR (2000) Is clinical examination an accurate indicator of raised intra-abdominal pressure in critically injured patients? Can J Surg 43:207–211
21. Greenhalgh DG, Warden GD (1994) The importance of intra-abdominal pressure measurements in burned children. J Trauma 36:685–690
22. Cheatham ML, White MW, Sagraves SG, Johnson JL, Block EF (2000) Abdominal perfusion pressure: a superior parameter in the assessment of intra-abdominal hypertension. J Trauma 49:621–626; discussion 626–627
23. Latenser BA, Kowal-Vern A, Kimball D, Chakrin A, Dujovny N (2002) A pilot study comparing percutaneous decompression with

decompressive laparotomy for acute abdominal compartment syndrome in thermal injury. J Burn Care Rehabil 23:190–195

24. Corcos AC, Sherman HF (2001) Percutaneous treatment of secondary abdominal compartment syndrome. J Trauma 51:1062–1064
25. Parra MW, Al-Khayat H, Smith HG, Cheatham ML (2006) Paracentesis for resuscitation-induced abdominal compartment syndrome: an alternative to decompressive laparotomy in the burn patient. J Trauma 60:1119–1121
26. Burlew CC, Moore EE, Biffl WL, Bensard DD, Johnson JL, Barnett CC (2012) One hundred percent fascial approximation can be achieved in the postinjury open abdomen with a sequential closure protocol. J Trauma Acute Care Surg 72:235–241
27. Feliciano DV, Mattox KL, Moore EE (2008) Trauma, 6th ed. McGraw-Hill Medical; New York, pp xxxi, 1430
28. Nathens AB, Rotstein OD, Marshall JC (1998) Tertiary peritonitis: clinical features of a complex nosocomial infection. World J Surg 22:158–163
29. Gracias VH, Braslow B, Johnson J, Pryor J, Gupta R, Reilly P et al (2002) Abdominal compartment syndrome in the open abdomen. Arch Surg 137:1298–1300
30. Johnson JW, Gracias VH, Schwab CW, Reilly PM, Kauder DR, Shapiro MB et al (2001) Evolution in damage control for exsanguinating penetrating abdominal injury. J Trauma 51:261–269; discussion 269–271
31. Sorrentino TA, Moore EE, Wohlauer MV, Biffl WL, Pieracci FM, Johnson JL et al (2012) Effect of damage control surgery on major abdominal vascular trauma. J Surg Res 177:320–325

Chapter 5
Surgical Treatment of Pelvic Fractures

Raffaele Pascarella, Luigi Rizzi, Claudio Castelli, and Rocco Politano

5.1 Introduction

Fracture of the pelvis ring is a rare lesion, 1–3 % of the traumatic skeletal lesion, that involves the three bones of the pelvis, nerves, vessels, and its viscera.

Initial management in trauma patients with pelvic fracture is aimed at saving life and identifying and treating life-threatening injuries in order of priority according to the ATLS rules. Mortality in pelvic fractures is reported to range between 9 and 20 % [1]. In hemodynamically unstable patients, mortality rate is generally up to 50 % due to a massive bleeding [2].

R. Pascarella • R. Politano
Department of Orthopedics and Trauma,
Ospedali Riuniti di Ancona,
Via Conca 71, Ancona 60126, Italy
e-mail: raffaele.pascarella@libero.it

L. Rizzi (✉) • C. Castelli
Department of Orthopedics and Trauma,
Ospedale Papa Giovanni XXIII, Piazza OMS 1, Bergamo 24127, Italy
e-mail: gigiriz@tin.it; ccastelli@hpg23.it

S. Di Saverio et al. (eds.), *Trauma Surgery*,
DOI 10.1007/978-88-470-5403-5_5, © Springer-Verlag Italia 2014

Definitive fixation of these lesions seeks to fix unstable lesions and to restore pelvic anatomy in order to avoid deformities and pain due to chronic instability and nonunion [3].

Planning the treatment in both emergency and definitive fixation is essential to classify the lesion.

5.2   Classification

The pelvis is a ring structure made up of three bones: the sacrum and the two innominates. The pelvic ring is formed by the connection of the sacrum to the innominate bones at the sacroiliac joints in the back and the symphysis pubis in the front. An important ligamentous complex also gives these joints strength and stability. Posteriorly interosseous, anterior and posterior sacroiliac ligaments are included with sacrotuberous, sacrospinous, and iliolumbar as connecting ligaments. Anteriorly, the opposed bony surface of the pubis is covered by hyaline cartilage and fibrous tissue.

The most recent is the AO classification that modifies the classification proposed by Tile in 1988 [4] and conforms with the nomenclature proposed by Muller and colleagues adopted by AO-ASIF groups [5]. Based on the integrity of the posterior sacroiliac complex and force direction of the injury, in this classification fractures are grouped into three groups, types A, B, or C, according to increased severity. Type A fractures are fractures with stability of the posterior ring. Type B includes fractures with partial posterior stability: these fractures are rotationally unstable but vertically stable. Type C unstable injury is a complete disruption of the posterior sacroiliac complex, involving vertical shear. Based on the anatomical lesions, many subgroups are also possible.

This classification is relevant not only for the management of the bony lesions but also for management of the patient particularly in emergency. All type A fractures have an intact stable pelvis, and treatment of bony injury does not affect the general condition of the patient. On the contrary, type B and type C fractures have partial and complete instability of the pelvis, respectively. Specific treatment of bony lesions has a major effect on the patient's outcome.

5.3   Surgical Treatment in Emergency

The polytrauma patient with pelvic ring injury is a very complex patient often hemodynamically unstable. In this condition, it is most important to determine the stability of the pelvic injury.

In a patient who is hemodynamically unstable with a stable pelvic ring injury, the saving of the life of the patient is the first priority. Because the pelvic ring injury is stable, it requires no further concern until such time as the patient becomes hemodynamically stable. The bleeding may be due to injury of the thoracic-abdominal organs, fractures of the limbs, open fractures, and vascular lesions of the pelvis. The control of bleeding is always a priority.

In a patient who is hemodynamically unstable with an unstable pelvic ring injury, the treatment of the pelvic lesion may be a part of the resuscitation procedure.

Intact pelvic ring encloses an anatomical space adapted to receive a significant amount of blood. Dalal et al. in 1989 [6], studying the behavior of the pressure/volume curve in the intact and injured pelvic ring, demonstrated that infusion of 5 l of liquid into the retroperitoneum of the intact pelvis increases the average pressure up to 30 mmHg and, in pelvic fracture infusion of 20 l of liquid, does not exceed the value of 35 mmHg. For this reason, stopping the bleeding in the injured pelvis is mechanically and dynamically impossible. Pelvic bleeding is caused by retroperitoneal venous plexus injuries in 80–85 % of cases and in the rest 15–20 % by arterial lesions [7].

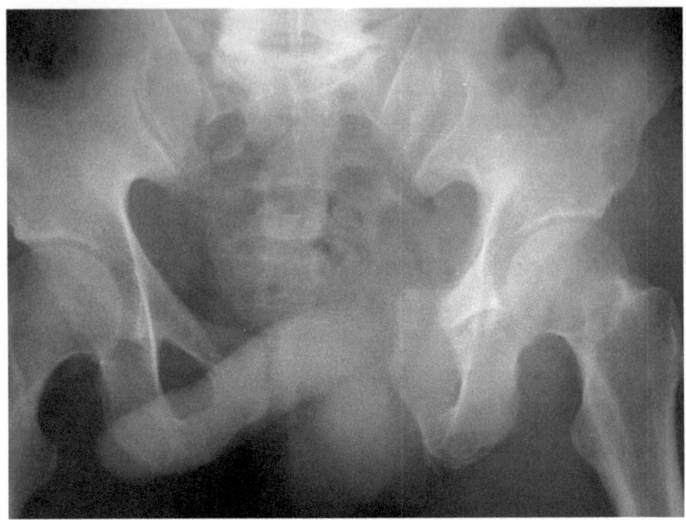

Fig. 5.1 Type C pelvic fracture to the left hemipelvis in a hemodynamically unstable 29-year-old man. Standard x-ray of the pelvis in the emergency room shows right sacral fracture, left sacroiliac joint dislocation, and symphysis pubis disruption

Standard x-ray of the pelvis in the emergency room is extremely useful in order to diagnose the pelvic fracture and to plan the stabilization [8]. Not all authors agreed on this behavior because it is argued that the quality and thus the diagnostic sensitivity of such x-ray are low (68 %) but nowadays are recognized as fundamental parts in the emergency diagnosis according to the ATLS rules (Fig. 5.1).

In case of an opening pelvic ring disruption, a reduction of the displaced hemipelvis should be performed immediately in the emergency room. The pelvic binder as a T-Pod is very simple to apply, is rapid, and stabilizes and reduces the pelvic volume. T-Pod must be removed within 24 h to avoid pressure sores on the patient.

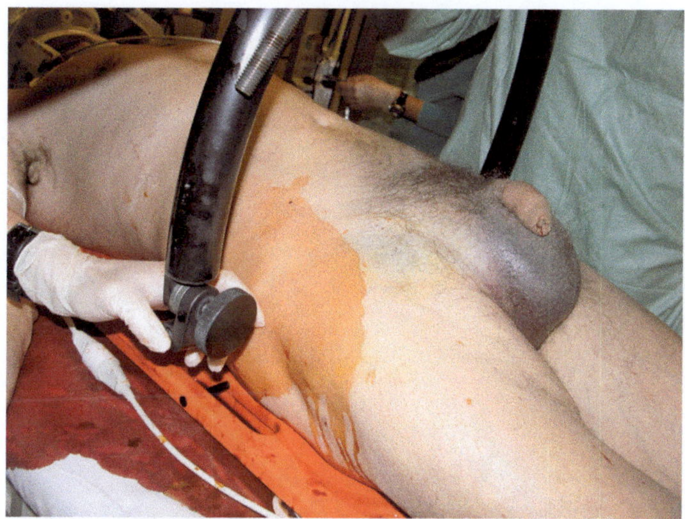

Fig. 5.2 The pelvic C-clamp is applied in the emergency room to stabilize the pelvis

Surgical treatment in the multiply injured patient in critical condition is performed with external fixation. External fixation of the pelvis has been demonstrated to temporarily stabilize an unstable pelvic fracture and effectively restore pelvic volume, thus improving survival. The application of external fixation has become a resuscitative tool that should be applied as soon as possible. Two main techniques are available to externally fix the unstable pelvic ring: external fixator and C-clamp. The external fixator is indicated in type B fractures, especially open-book type injuries. Pins (at least two on each side of the pelvis) are placed into the iliac crest behind the anterior-superior iliac spine. This placement is safe and easy, and an image intensifier is not necessary.

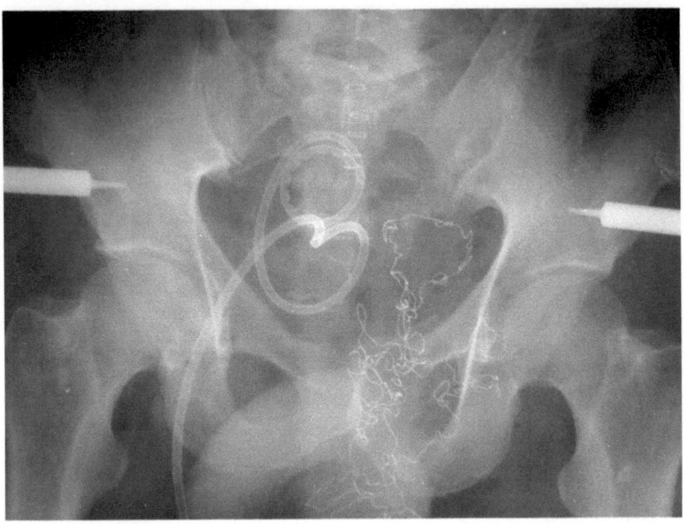

Fig. 5.3 Standard x-ray of the pelvis after application of the clamp shows the restoration of the pelvic ring and stabilization of the patient, who survived after laparotomy

An absolute indication for external fixation is a severe open pelvic fracture with abdominal lesion that requires colostomy in order to prevent serious infection of the wound and promote rapid healing.

In unstable type C injuries, the pelvic C-clamp (Fig. 5.2) is recommended. The pelvic C-clamp, introduced by Reinhold Ganz [9] 20 years ago, is a device with two pins applied posteriorly in the area of the pelvis lateral to the sacroiliac joints. The pelvic C-clamp is applied quickly, about 15 min, and stabilizes the pelvis, decreasing effectively its diameter (Fig. 5.3). Most importantly, it does not interfere with the ability to perform subsequent laparotomy or other surgical procedure. The pelvic C-clamp may not be used in the presence of iliac wing fracture [9]. Pelvic C-clamp must be removed within 72 h because it is no longer useful and starts to mobilize.

5.4 Definitive Surgical Treatment

When the patient's general status permits type B and type C fractures, open reduction and internal fixation (ORIF) of all fractures and joint reconstruction have to be performed [3]. Nonoperative treatment of displaced and unstable pelvic fractures results in a high percentage of bad outcomes with deformities and pain due to chronic instability and nonunion. The best time for an ORIF of the pelvic fracture is soon as possible depending of the patient's general status. Most of these fractures are treated at the end of the first week and during the second one when hematoma is not yet organized and fracture reduction is still easy.

According to the AO classification, type B fractures are treated definitively with an anterior fixation, while type C fractures need an anterior and/or posterior internal fixation depending on anatomical lesions.

For the symphysis disruption, we used open reduction and plate fixation through the Pfannenstiel approach. In sacroiliac dislocation and in sacral fracture, our preferred surgical option is iliosacral screws that can be done with open or closed techniques. Plate fixation is indicated in iliac wing fractures performed usually through the ilioinguinal approach.

The benefits of ORIF are represented by the anatomical reduction and biomechanically more stable fixation of the fracture that allow early mobilization, shorter hospitalization, and improved outcomes.

5.5 Conclusions

Surgical treatment of pelvic fracture is different when performed in emergency or as a definitive treatment. Classification is relevant for the management of these bony lesions that must only be done by experienced surgeons who can operate safety in appropriate environment. Better clinical results are related to the more stability of the fixation of the posterior pelvic ring. Anatomical reduction of the pelvic ring and internal fixation of the disruption of the pelvis is the gold standard in the treatment of these lesions.

References

1. Moreno C, Moore EE, Rosenberger A, Cleveland HC (1986) Hemorrhage associated with major pelvic fracture: a multispecialty challenge. J Trauma 26(11):987–994
2. Pohlemann T, Bosch U, Gansslen A, Tscherne H (1994) The Hannover experience in management of pelvic fractures. Clin Orthop 305:69–80
3. Matta JM, Saucedo T (1989) Internal fixation of pelvic ring fractures. Clin Orthop 242:83–97
4. Tile M (1988) Pelvic ring fractures: should they be fixed? J Bone Joint Surg Br 70(1):1–12
5. Muller ME, Allgower M, Schneider R, Willenegger H (1990) Manual of internal fixation, 3rd edn. Springer, Berlin
6. Dalal SA, Burgess AR, Siegel JH, Young JW, Brumback RJ, Poka A, Dunham CM, Gens D, Bathon H (1989) Pelvis fracture in multiple trauma: classification by mechanism is key to pattern of organ injury, resuscitative requirements and outcome. J Trauma 29(7):981–1000
7. Brown JJ, Greene FL, Mc Millin RD (1984) Vascular injuries associated with pelvic fractures. Am Surg 50(3):150–154
8. Obaid AK, Barleben A, Porral D, Lush S, Cinat M (2006) Utility of plain film pelvic radiographs in blunt trauma patients in the emergency department. Am Surg 72:951–954
9. Ganz R, Krushell RJ, Jakob RP, Kuffer J (1991) The antishock pelvic clamp. Clin Orthop 267:71–78

Chapter 6
Surgery of the Cervical Spine Trauma

Federico De Iure and Luca Amendola

6.1 General Consideration

6.1.1 Epidemiology

Injuries of the spinal column should be suspected in all cases of high-energy trauma (20 % of all polytrauma cases [1]). Motor vehicle accidents (MVA) are the most frequent cause of severe spine trauma (49 %), followed by falls from a height (20 %). About 50 % of all severe spine injuries are not diagnosed or underestimated in the prehospital setting, especially in unconscious patients.

F. De Iure (✉) • L. Amendola
Spine Surgery Department, Trauma Center – Ospedale
Maggiore-Bologna, Largo Bartolo Nigrisoli 2,
Bologna 40100, Italy
e-mail: federico.deiure@ausl.bologna.it; luca.amendola@yahoo.it

S. Di Saverio et al. (eds.), *Trauma Surgery*,
DOI 10.1007/978-88-470-5403-5_6, © Springer-Verlag Italia 2014

6.1.2 Preoperative Management

Polytraumatized/unconscious patients require in-line immobilization of the cervical spine by stiff collar and of the thoracolumbar spine by spine board or vacuum mattress. There is no scientific evidence of benefit by preoperative high-dose corticosteroid infusion; therefore, this practice should be abandoned.

6.1.3 Imaging

Multislice CT scan is the gold standard for spine clearance in polytrauma patients. MRI is mandatory in spinal cord injuries whenever the neurologic level is different from the level of the injury detected by CT or if no bony injury is found. Spine injuries not requiring surgery in emergency should anyway complete imaging by MRI to evaluate the posterior ligament complex integrity and/or disk disruption and/or epidural hematoma.

6.1.4 Surgical Timing

Provided life-threatening injuries have been excluded or treated, spine stabilization should be performed as soon as possible. Spine stabilization within 72 h, especially in polytrauma patients (ISS 18 or above), greatly decreases both the rate of general complications and the length of stay in ICU [2]. In case of neurologic damage, decompression and stabilization should be delivered immediately.

6.2 Upper Cervical Spine Injuries

Upper cervical spine morphology is peculiar compared to the subaxial vertebral column. During the embryo development, C0, C1, and C2 sclerotomes form the odontoid process of C2

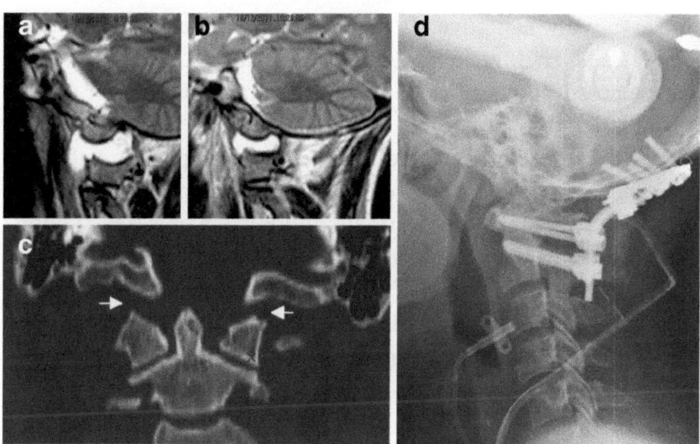

Fig. 6.1 Occipitocervical dislocation following car accident. Hyperintense signal on T2-weighted MRI showing blood inside C0-C1 left (**a**) and right (**b**) joints. Frontal plane CT scan (**c**) showing increased distance between occipital condyles and C1 articular masses (*white arrows*). Occipitocervical posterior fusion on post-op x-rays (**d**)

which, in adult life, will act as a fulcrum allowing nearly 50 % of the rotation of the head above the trunk. This particular anatomy explains the various patterns of UCS injuries that are described below.

Occipital condyles fractures may follow head injuries, and their morphology is described in Anderson and Montesano classification [3]. They are generally stable and can be treated by either stiff collar or halo jacket. Type III fractures are likely to be unstable and require an occipitocervical fusion if a residual instability is detected after conservative treatment.

Occipitocervical dissociation is frequently fatal. The most frequent pattern is the anterior translocation of the occipital condyle relative to the atlantal lateral masses. In surviving patients, occipitocervical fusion is mandatory as the injury is critically unstable and both collar and halo jacket can only be used as temporary stabilization devices (Fig. 6.1).

Atlas burst fracture (Jefferson's fractures) with minimal displacement of the lateral masses is considered stable and treated conservatively as above. If the displacement exceeds 10 mm, then a transverse ligament and/or alar ligament disruption must be suspected. In case of late instability, then a C0-C2 or C1-C2 fusion is required [4].

Odontoid fractures were classified in tree types by Anderson and D'Alonzo according to its site (apex, mid-part, basis). Anterior screwing is the treatment of choice in axis type 2 odontoid fracture in young patients [5]. It guarantees the highest rate of healing, preserving C1-C2 motility. Nevertheless the rate of healing may decrease rapidly in the elderly, so some authors perform a C1-C2 posterior fusion as first surgery in these patients. Type 1 and type 3 fractures can be treated conservatively by halo jacket or stiff collar.

C2 traumatic spondylolysis (Hangman fracture) can be treated conservatively in case of minimal displacement and without signs of C2-C3 disk injury (types I and IIa) [6]. Anterior discectomy and fusion is required in case of anterior dislocation following disk disruption. Unilateral or bilateral facet dislocation is rarely seen in these injuries and should be reduced and fixed by posterior approach (type III).

C1-C2 rotatory dislocation was classified by Fielding and Hawking [7] and may follow high-energy trauma in adult patients. This situation is more frequently seen in children because of their skeletal immaturity, even following low-energy trauma, and should be treated immediately by closed reduction (traction and counter rotation) and collar immobilization for 3 weeks. In adults, or also in children if diagnosis is delayed more than 2 weeks, reduction becomes difficult and immobilization is delivered by halo jacket for a longer period. In selected cases, when reduction by external maneuvers becomes impossible, then posterior open reduction and fixation is performed.

Atlas transverse ligament rupture is not frequent and is generally accompanied by head injuries. For this reason diagnosis is frequently delayed and revealed by a C1-C2 late instability on the sagittal plane. As spontaneous healing of purely ligamentous

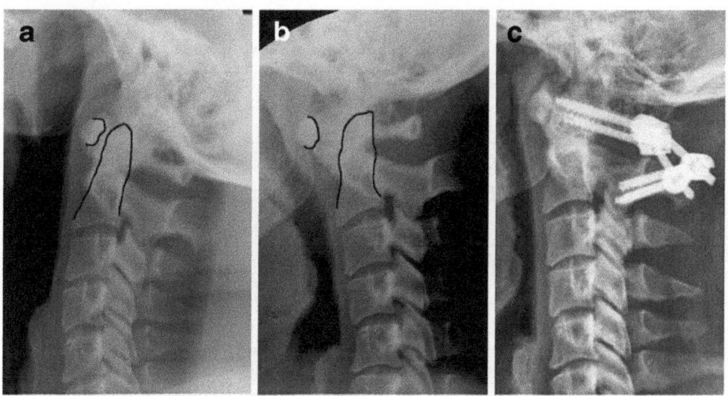

Fig. 6.2 C1-C2 sagittal instability due to transverse ligament injury. The distance between odontoid and atlas anterior arch increases in flexion (**b**) compared to extension (**a**). A C1-C2 posterior fusion is performed (**c**)

injury is unlikely to happen, then the treatment of choice is a C1-C2 fusion (Fig. 6.2).

6.3   Lower Cervical Spine (LCS) Injuries (T1)

No worldwide accepted classification is found in the literature for these injuries, and no classification suits all the possible injuries a spine surgeon may encounter in his/her professional life. Most of the following consideration are drawn by Claude Argenson's works [8, 9]. LCS injuries are divided in compression (type A), flexion-extension (type B), and rotation (type C) according to the possible pathogenesis. It is easy to keep in mind and can be easily related with radiologic evidence giving an immediate indication for surgery (Table 6.1).

Simple anterior wedging (A1) of a LCS vertebral body can be treated conservatively by halo jacket or stiff collar whenever local kyphosis is less than 15°. Greater deformities may require surgical correction and fusion.

Table 6.1 Indications for lower cervical spine injuries treatment are reported according to Argensons' classification

| | Severity | | |
Type	1	2	3
A (compression)	CT	ACF	ACF
B (flexion-extension)	CT	ADF	ADF+PF
C (rotation)	CT or ADF	CT or ADF	ADF or PF+ADF

CT conservative treatment, *ACF* anterior corpectomy and fusion, *ADF* anterior discectomy and fusion, *PF* posterior reduction and fusion

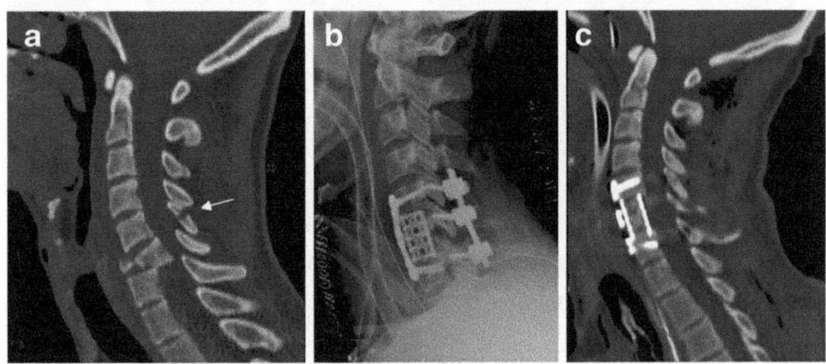

Fig. 6.3 C6 "teardrop" fracture with posterior dislocation of the cervical spine above the injury (**a**) due to a motorbike accident. The spinal canal is narrowed and the posterior elements are also involved (*white arrow*). Standard x-ray shows realignment of the spine after C6 corpectomy and double approach fixation (**b**). The spinal canal is fully decompressed on post-op CT scan (**c**)

"Teardrop" fractures (A3) and "burst" fractures (A2) involve the anterior column, are frequently associated with neurologic damage, and require anterior corpectomy and fusion by plate and tricortical graft or titanium mesh. In case of massive disruption of the posterior ligament complex, a posterior short fixation should be carried on in adjunct (Fig. 6.3).

Moderate sprain injuries (B1) due to flexion-extension trauma do not require surgical treatment. If a disk rupture is diagnosed in addition, then anterior discectomy and fusion is the treatment of choice even in case sagittal alignment is preserved (B2). "Bilateral facets dislocation" and "traumatic spondylolis-thesis" (B3) can be reduced and fixed by anterior approach following discectomy. In both cases, but especially in traumatic spondylolisthesis, we suggest a posterior fixation in addition.

Rotation injuries are characterized by a disk injury associated with a "unilateral facet fracture" (C1 type) or an "articular mass fracture dislocation" (C2 type) or a "unilateral facet dislocation" (C3 type). A moderate anterior dislocation of the CS above the injured disk is the common pattern. Anterior discectomy and fusion is the treatment of choice. Unilateral facet dislocation can be irreducible by external maneuvers; thus, a posterior open reduction before anterior fusion can be necessary. Conservative treatment can be attempted (C1 and C2 type) in case sagittal alignment is preserved, assuming no disk injury is associated, but a close radiologic follow-up is then mandatory.

Fractures and dislocations of the LCS in ankylotic spine are generally seen in the elderly. Additional injuries in the thoracic or lumbar spine are frequently found. Therefore a preoperative radiologic study of the whole spine is mandatory. Due to the calcified disks, the cervical spine behaves as a fractured long bone and the injury is very unstable. Neurologic damage is frequently present (generally a central cord syndrome), and decompression can be achieved indirectly by spine realignment during surgery. Due to osteoporosis, we recommend posterior oversized fixation (tree level above and below the injury at least).

References

1. Schinkel C, Frangen TM, Kmetic A, Andress H-J, Muhr G (2007) Spinal fractures in multiply injured patients. An analysis of the German Trauma Society's Trauma Register. Unfallchirurg 110:946–952

2. Rutges JP, Oner FC, Leenen LP (2007) Timing of thoracic and lumbar fracture fixation in spinal injuries: a systematic review of neurologic and clinical outcome. Eur Spine J 16:579–587
3. Anderson PA, Montesano PX (1988) Morphology and treatment of occipital condyle fractures. Spine 13:731–736
4. Spence KF Jr, Decker S, Sell KW (1970) Bursting atlantal fracture associated with rupture of the transverse ligament. J Bone Joint Surg 52:543–549
5. Anderson LD, D'Alonzo RT (1974) Fractures of the odontoid process of the axis. J Bone Joint Surg 56 A:1663–1674
6. Levine AM, Edwards CC (1985) The management of traumatic spondylolisthesis of the axis. J Bone Joint Surg Am 67:217–226
7. Fielding JW, Hawkins RJ (1977) Atlanto-axial rotatory fixation. J Bone Joint Surg 59:37–44
8. Argenson C, de Peretti F, Ghabris A et al (1997) Classification of lower cervical spine injuries. Eur J Orthop Surg Traumatol 7:215–229
9. Argenson C, de Peretti F, Ghabris A et al (2012) A scheme for the classification of lower cervical spine injuries. Maitrise-orthop. http://www.maitrise-orthop.com/corpusmaitri/orthopaedic/mo61_spine_injury_class/spine_injury.shtml. Accessed 2 Jan 2012

Chapter 7
Surgery of the Thoracolumbar Spine Trauma

Ralf H. Gahr and Matthias Spalteholz

Fifty percent of all relevant thoracic and lumbar spine injuries are located within the thoracolumbar junction T12–L2, due to the biomechanical transition from the stiff and rigid thoracic kyphosis to the highly mobile adjacent lordosis of the lumbar spine. In mid-thoracic spine the spinal canal is very narrow in relation to the spinal cord. Already a compromise of the spinal canal of less than 20 % may lead to higher degrees of spinal cord injury. At the level of the thoracolumbar junction, the reserve space around the spinal cord is relatively wide so that even a spinal canal compromise of up to 40 % does not automatically lead to neurological deficits. The indication for surgery is dependent on neurological symptoms, mechanical instability, and deformity. According to the 3-column model of Denis, injuries of the anterior, middle and posterior column are classified [1]. The anterior column ensures load bearing while the posterior column acts as a dorsal tension band.

R.H. Gahr (✉) • M. Spalteholz
Traumazentrum "St. Georg" Leipzig,
Klinik für Unfallchirurgie und Orthopädie,
Delitzscherstr. 141, Leipzig 04129, Germany
e-mail: ralf.gahr@sanktgeorg.de; matthias.spalteholtz@sanktgeorg.de

S. Di Saverio et al. (eds.), *Trauma Surgery*,
DOI 10.1007/978-88-470-5403-5_7, © Springer-Verlag Italia 2014

7.1   Nonoperative Treatment

Functional treatment with pain-adapted mobilization and muscle training is recommended for A1.1, A1.2, and A2.1, A2.2 fractures with intact adjacent discs. In general, the limiting factor is a kyphosis of less than 20° and a reduction of height of less than 50 %.

Minimal invasive operative techniques have widened the spectrum of surgical treatment. The indication for surgery is also influenced by national specifics (legal issues, social security).

7.2   Surgical Treatment

Surgical treatment depends mainly on the type of fracture, potential spinal cord involvement, and additional adverse effects (polytrauma, morbidity, age, bone quality) (Figs. 7.1, 7.2, 7.3, 7.4, 7.5, 7.6, and 7.7).

7.2.1   Type A Fractures

7.2.1.1   A1.1, A1.2 (>20° Kyphosis), A1.3

BAER (balloon-assisted end plate reduction, that is, kyphoplasty plus short segment minimal invasive dorsal stabilization, intravertebral cage system).

7.2.1.2   A2.3

Bisegmental anterior spinal fusion (partial vertebrectomy/cage plus anterior plate or dual-rod system). High risk of intrusion of disc material into vertebral body with resulting vertebral nonunion.

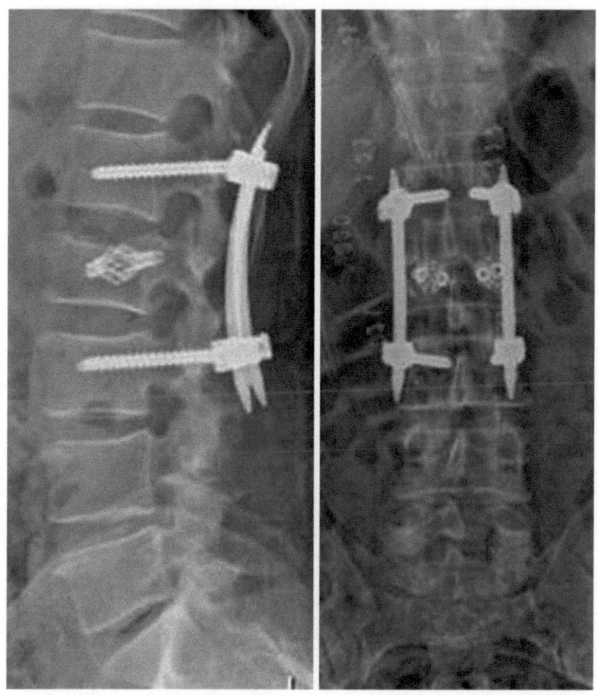

Fig. 7.1 Fractured L2 (A3.1). Posterior bisegmental instrumentation and L2 reduction by expandable cage

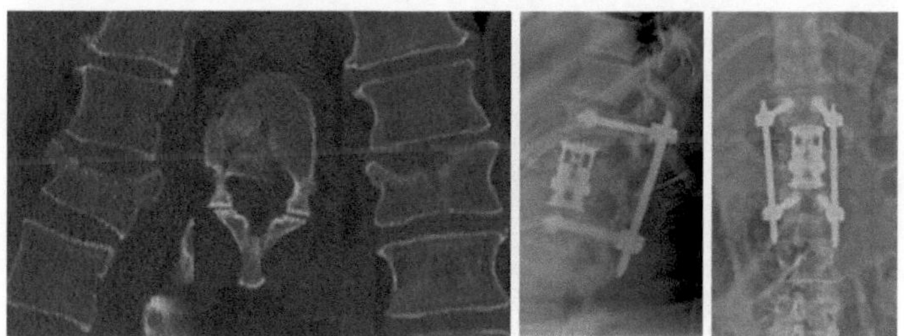

Fig. 7.2 Fractured L1 (A3.2). Cement-augmented posterior stabilization, anterior subtotal corporectomy, and cage reconstruction

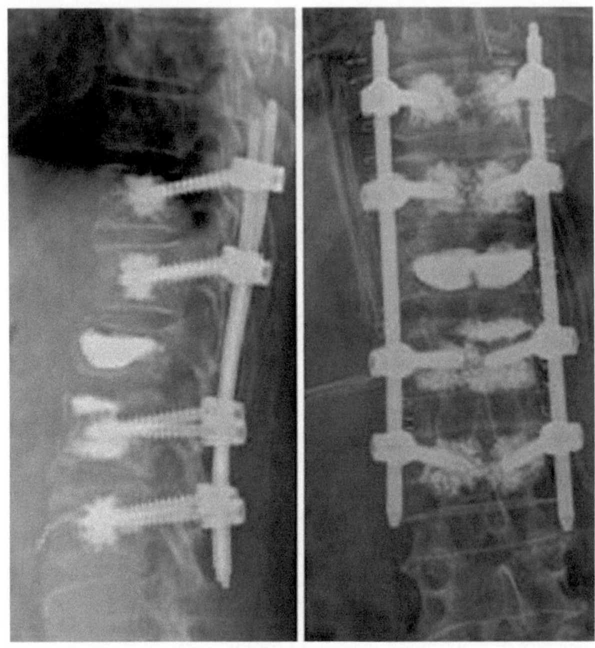

Fig. 7.3 L1 fracture in osteoporotic bone (B2). Augmented posterior long-segment stabilization and kyphoplasty

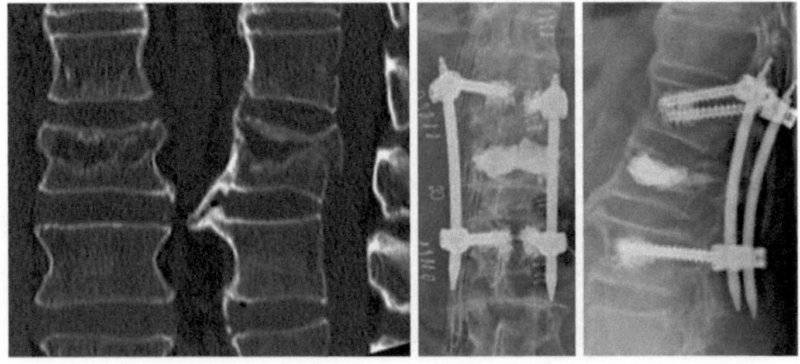

Fig. 7.4 L1 fracture (A3.1). Kyphoplasty (BAER) and augmented posterior bisegmental stabilization

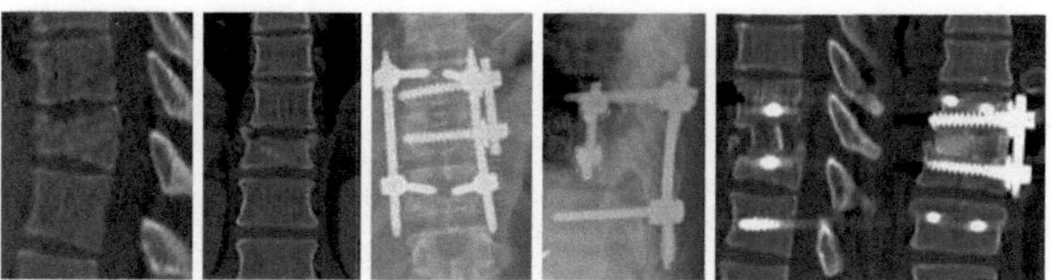

Fig. 7.5 Fractured Th11 (A3.1). Posterior bisegmental instrumentation and anterior monosegmental reconstruction with iliac chip

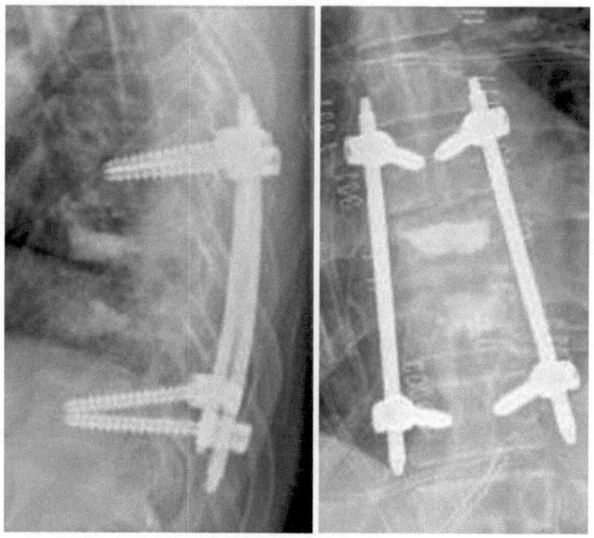

Fig. 7.6 Th 8 and Th 9 fracture (A3.1). Posterior stabilization and kyphoplasty with resorbable bone substitute

7.2.1.3 A3.1, A3.2

Short segment minimal invasive dorsal stabilization (plus BAER).

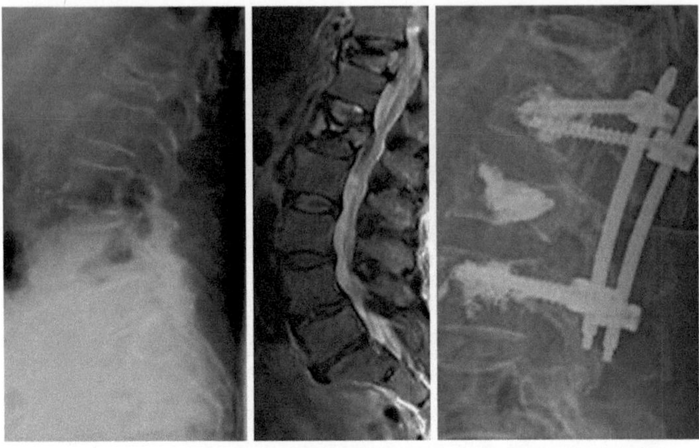

Fig. 7.7 Osteoporotic L1 fracture (A1.3). Kyphoplasty (BAER) and augmented posterior bisegmental stabilization

7.2.1.4   A3.3

In polytrauma, primary minimal invasive dorsal stabilization. Canal compromise or spinal cord involvement requires immediate anterior decompression and reconstruction of the anterior column (expendable cage).

Secondary reconstruction of the anterior column (BAER, if sufficient, in older patients; intravertebral expandable cage system including ruptured adjacent discs).

7.2.2   *Type B Fractures*

Posterior reduction and long-segment stabilization (dorsal construct acts as tension band), additional ventral stabilization, and reconstruction according to the needs of the ventral A component.

7.2.3   *Type C Fractures*

Highest degree of instability; usually require dorsoventral reduction and stabilization.

Reference

1. Denis F (1983) The three column spine and is significance in the classification of acute thoracolumbar spinal injuries. Spine 8:817–831

Chapter 8
Trauma Surgery of the Extremities

Ralf H. Gahr and Matthias Spalteholz

Isolated fractures of the extremities are rarely life threatening [1]. However, stabilization of long bone injuries is obligatory within the first 24 h. Open fractures, compartment syndromes, and vascular and neural injuries require emergency treatment within 6 h [2].

In polytraumatized patients extremity surgery is no longer focussed on early total repair but on damage control. ATLS criteria were transferred to trauma surgery algorithms ("Treat first what kills first").

Primary external fixation is the tool for the stabilization of bone and joints in emergency situations; also when primary internal fixation is contraindicated, e.g., higher-grade open and closed fractures, external fixation is the treatment of choice (short operative time, minimal intraoperative hemorrhage). Definite internal osteosynthesis should be performed electively after 4–5 days. Definitive treatment by external fixation is also

R.H. Gahr (✉) • M. Spalteholz
Traumazentrum "St. Georg" Leipzig,
Klinik für Unfallchirurgie und Orthopädie,
Delitzscherstr. 141, Leipzig 04129, Germany
e-mail: ralf.gahr@sanktgeorg.de; mathias.spalteholtz@sanktgeorg.de

S. Di Saverio et al. (eds.), *Trauma Surgery*,
DOI 10.1007/978-88-470-5403-5_8, © Springer-Verlag Italia 2014

feasible, but there is high risk of pin tract infection, malalignment, and pseudarthrosis [3]. Even in emergency surgery, the primary external construct should always anatomically correct and biomechanically stable.

Because of their potential long-term disabilities, the following injuries should receive primary definite treatment even in polytrauma, whenever possible: medial femoral neck fractures in younger patients (<60), hip dislocations, dislocated talus fractures, and irreducible dislocations [4].

8.1 Upper Extremity Injuries

8.1.1 Shoulder Dislocations

The most common dislocation/luxation (80–90 % are anterior, about 5 % each posterior or inferior dislocations). Anterior dislocations usually result from forced external rotation and abduction. Posterior dislocations are frequently associated with epileptic seizures and electrical accidents. People under 40 years typically show lesions of the capsular-ligamentous complex. Rotator cuff lesions have high incidence in older patients (>60 years) [5]. Bankart fractures and labral lesions must be stabilized electively. Sometimes recurrent posttraumatic luxations are due to Hill-Sachs lesions. The impacted bone should be elevated and the defect relined. Several reduction techniques have been reported, e.g., by Hippocrates, Kocher, Arlt, and Stimson.

8.1.2 Humeral Head Fractures

Proximal humeral fractures in low-energy accidents are typical for elderly patients with osteoporosis. In younger people these fractures are usually caused by high-energy traumata like road traffic accidents. Proximal humeral fractures are classified by Neer [6]: four main parts, six fracture types. The therapy depends on the fracture type and the extent of displacement. Surgery is recommended when the head angulation is greater than 25° and the displacement of the tubercula is greater than 5 mm. Major fragment displacement may result in concomitant axillar nerve injury or secondary avascular necrosis of the humeral head.

Isolated fractures of the tubercula may be fixed by cannulated screws. 2- and 3-part fractures as well as 4-part fractures in young patients are treated with open (or closed) reduction and internal locking plate fixation. In elderly patients there is a growing tendency for primary arthroplasty in 4-part injuries.

8.1.3   Humeral Shaft Fractures

Humeral shaft fractures have been the domain of conservative treatment (functional bracing) until the early 1990s. The last two decades have seen a gradual change towards operative treatment, due to the development of unreamed locking nails and locking plate systems as well as a change in patient's demands.

Standard procedure is either orthograde (more distal diaphyseal fractures) or retrograde (more proximal diaphyseal fractures, obese patients) intramedullary nailing. Plate osteosynthesis is required in long-comminuted fractures or whenever open reduction/radial nerve revision is necessary.

Depending on the fracture localization, the following approaches are used: extended anterolateral approach for proximal fractures and triceps split (Henry) for distal fractures.

Secondary radial nerve paralysis is an indication for nerve revision.

8.1.4 *Distal Humeral Fractures*

Extraarticular, partial intraarticular, and intraarticular fractures are distinguished. The risk of neurovascular damage rises with the extent of the fracture displacement. Especially the development of a compartment syndrome must be recognized (Volkmann's contracture in children). In case of critical soft tissue conditions, open fractures, and compartment syndromes, a joint spanning external fixator should be used for primary stabilization. The operative procedure depends on the fracture type. Compression screw fixation is indicated in A1, B1, and B2 fractures. Open reduction and internal small fragment screw fixation are used in B3 fractures. In case of severe articular surface destruction, primary total elbow replacement may be considered in older patients [7]. A2 and A3 fractures are fixed by anatomically preformed plates (ORIF). Open reduction and internal plate fixation is necessary in all C-type fractures: The joint block is primarily reconstructed and stabilized by K-wires or screws and then fixed to the proximal fragment by anatomically preformed (locking) plates. Maximal stability results from positioning the plates rectangularly to each other [8]. A dorsal approach without (triceps on) or with olecranon osteotomy provides sufficient joint exploration. The intraoperative identification and protection of the ulnar nerve is obligatory. The goal of surgery is the anatomical reconstruction of the articular planes, early mobilization, and the prevention of secondary arthrofibrosis and functional disability. Indometacin is recommended for 14 days to avoid heterotopic ossification (Figs. 8.1 and 8.2).

8.1.5 *Elbow Luxations*

The forearm most frequently dislocates posteriorly (posterolateral, posteromedial). Anterior dislocations are rare. The evaluation of the neurovascular status is mandatory. After reduction in analgo-sedation, the elbow should be immobilized (cast, >90°).

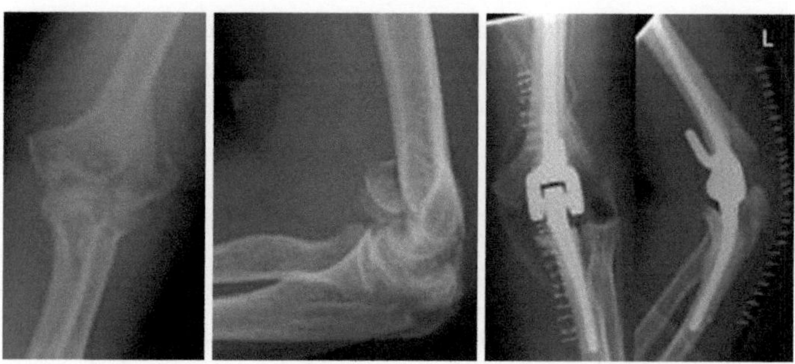

Fig. 8.1 Type B 3 fracture and primary total elbow replacement

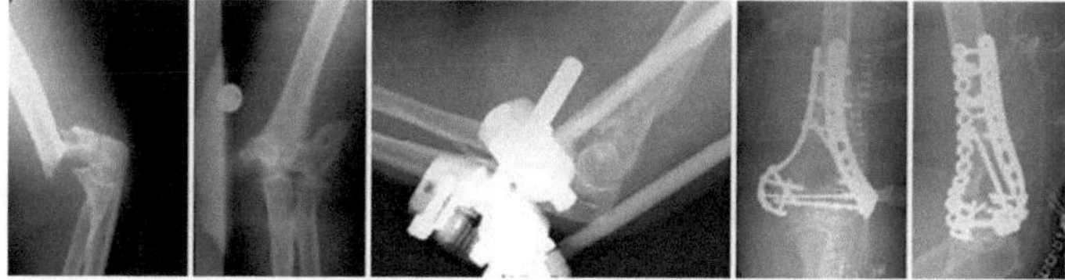

Fig. 8.2 Transcondylar humerus fracture (C2). Primary closed reduction and external fixator stabilization. Secondary open reduction and internal (anatomical) plate fixation after soft tissue consolidation

The following treatment depends on the dynamic and static elbow stability. In case of biomechanical joint stability (coronoid intact), the therapy is nonoperative. Dynamic instabilities and coronoid fractures should be stabilized after soft tissue consolidation.

8.2 Proximal Forearm Fractures

8.2.1 Olecranon Fractures

Olecranon fractures are classified by Schatzker [9]. These fractures are tensile-loaded fractures; therefore tension band wiring is the standard procedure for simple fractures. For the stability it is very important to anchor the wires in the opposite corticalis. Proximal transverse fractures may be fixed by cancellous compression screws. Plate fixation is used for comminuted fractures (LCDCP/LCP).

8.2.2 Radial Head Fractures

The treatment is based on the Mason classification. Type 1 fractures are treated nonoperatively. Type 2 fractures are indication for open reduction and internal mini-screw fixation. Closed reduction and titanium elastic nail fixation may be performed in displaced fractures of the radial neck (Metaizeau technique) [10]. Open reduction and mini-plate fixation are used in type 3 fractures. Radial head resection is an option in comminuted factures. The radial head replacement is necessary in case of instability of the lateral column to prevent a proximal migration of the radius and in case of laceration of the interosseous membrane (Essex-Lopresti fracture).

8.2.3 Forearm Shaft Fractures

Ulna and radial parry fractures are distinguished from forearm fractures. In general nonoperative therapy is possible. However, surgery offers the opportunity of functional treatment. The classic forearm fracture is an absolutely indication for surgery. A2 and A3 fractures have to be fixed under compression with LCDC plates to avoid pseudarthroses. Locking plate systems are used to stabilize A1, B, and C fractures. The stabilization starts with the ulna fracture by using a medial, intermuscular approach. Thompson's approach is the standard approach for radius shaft fractures [11]. In case of very proximal radius fractures, the Henry approach is recommended [12]. It is very important to protect the profund branch of the radial nerve. Unimpeded pro- and supination should be documented after plate fixation.

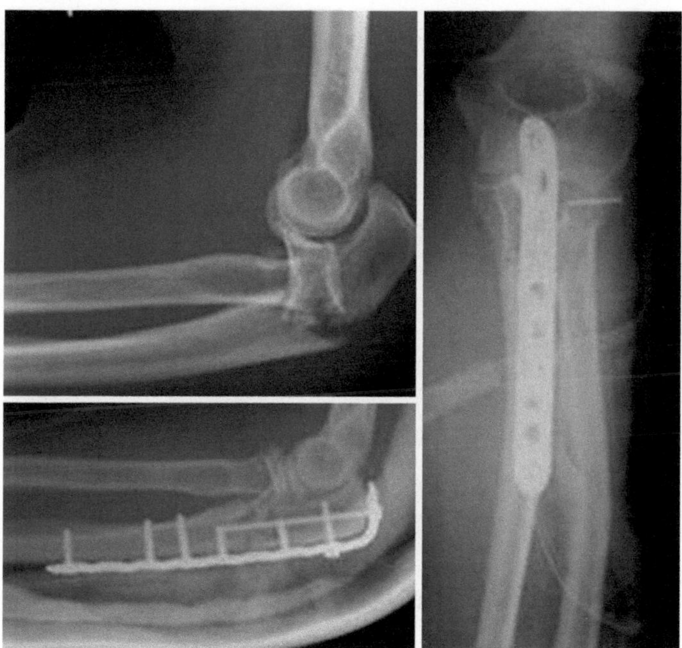

Fig. 8.3 Monteggia-like lesion. Open reduction and plate fixation of the ulna. Mini-screw fixation of the radial head

8.2.4   Monteggia Fractures

Fracture of the proximal third of the ulna with dislocation of the radial head.

Bado describes four types, depending on the dislocation of the radial head. The Monteggia-like lesion describes an additional radial head fracture. Usually, the anatomical reduction of the ulna fracture leads to a spontaneous radial head reduction. LC and LCDC plates are used for internal fixation. The humeroradial joint should be explored in case of instability, and the annular ligament should be reconstructed (Fig. 8.3).

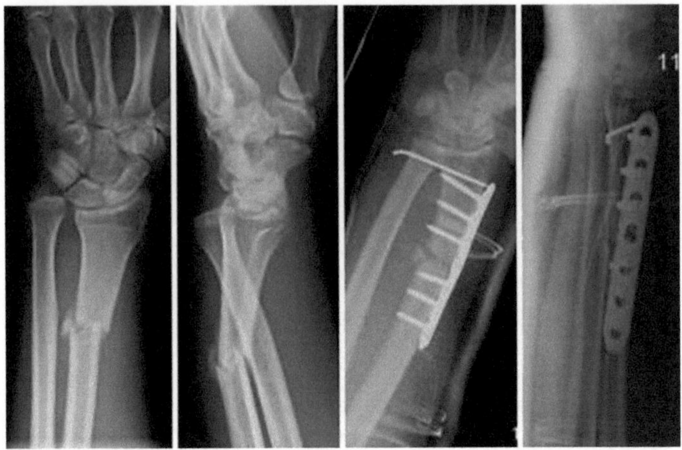

Fig. 8.4 Galeazzi fracture. Open reduction and internal radius plate fixation. K-wire transfixation of the DRUJ

8.2.5 Galeazzi fractures

Fracture of the radius shaft with dislocation of the ulnar head. Open reduction and internal plate fixation (LCDCP) of the radius lead to the reduction of the distal radioulnar joint (DRUJ). In case of DRUJ instability, temporary transfixation may be necessary (K-wires and long arm cast for 8 weeks) (Fig. 8.4).

8.2.6 Essex-Lopresti Fractures

The Essex-Lopresti lesion represents a complex distorsion injury of the wrist, comparable to the mechanism of a Maisonneuve fracture. The Essex-Lopresti fracture is a combination of DRUJ dislocation, laceration of the interosseous membrane, and radial head fracture [13]. These unstable injuries need surgery: temporary transfixation of the distal radioulnar joint, internal fixation of the radial head, and in case of comminuted fractures a radial head replacement.

8.2.7 Distal Radial Fractures

Distal radius fractures are the most common fractures (25 %), frequently seen in osteoporotic patients. Depending of the position of the hand during a fall, different fracture types are distinguished. The aim of the treatment is to restore the 3 columns of the wrist anatomically (reconstruction of the Böhler's angle). Palmar locking plate fixation is recommended for type A2, A3, B2, B3, C1, and 2.3 fractures. Chauffeur fractures (B1) are fixed by compression screws. The intrafocal (Kapandji) or extrafocal (Willenegger) K-wire osteosynthesis may be used in A2 fractures or in critical soft tissue conditions, when open reduction is not possible. K-wires are also used in addition to plates or external fixators in case of destruction of the articulating surface. Bridging external fixators are useful in osteoporotic-comminuted fractures, precarious soft tissue conditions, high-grade open fractures, and polytraumatized patients. Additional injuries like SL—dissociations, displaced fractures of the base of the ulna styloid, and TFCC—and DRUJ instabilities require additional surgery.

8.3 Lower Limb Injuries

8.3.1 Femoral Head Fractures

Fractures of the femoral head (frequently combined with dorsal hip dislocation or femoral neck fractures) are the result of a high-energy trauma (e.g., dash board injury). The Pipkin classification describes 4 types [14]. The indication for open reduction and internal screw fixation of type 1 fractures depends on the extent of head destruction, fragment displacement, and impingement. Surgery is indicated in all type 2–4 cases. The main complications resulting from femoral head fractures are AVN of the femoral head, heterotopic ossification, and secondary coxarthrosis.

8.3.2   *Femoral Neck Fractures*

In the times of conservative treatment, femoral neck fractures had an extremely high mortality rate due to immobilization-related complications (DVT, pulmonary embolism, pneumonia).

Even today femoral neck fractures of the elderly show 1-year mortality of up to 25 %.

The Pauwels classification, defining the degree of instability based on the angle between the fracture and the horizontal plane, was used to identify stable fractures, which could be treated conservatively, and unstable fractures, which needed surgery, have become obsolete, as most fractures today are treated with primary hip replacement. The Garden classification considers the extent of the displacement and is used to estimate the prognosis of the fracture regarding the risk of nonunion and AVN.

Because of the compromised blood supply of the femoral head, only minimal displaced neck fractures in younger patients stand a chance of unimpaired fracture healing. These fractures should be reduced and fixed with cannulated screws preferably within the first 6 h to ensure best results. Operative decompression of the hip joint is controversial.

Hip replacement is recommended within 24–36 h. Studies did not show any significant differences between the use of bipolar prostheses or total hip replacement [15].

8.3.3 Trochanteric Fractures

According to the AO classification, trochanteric fractures are classified into stable and unstable fractures. There are three types of instabilities: mediolateral, craniocaudal, and rotational instability. The posteromedial support (lesser trochanter defect) and the involvement of the subtrochanteric region are crucial for the stability. The mini-open reduction and extramedullary stabilization (e.g., by DHS) may be used for stable trochanteric fractures (31A1). Intramedullary nailing with cephalomedullary nails has become the gold standard for all types of intertrochanteric and subtrochanteric fractures, as these nails are suitable for both stable and unstable fractures.

Fixation of the lesser trochanter is not necessary. In displaced fractures with involvement of the subtrochanteric region, open reduction and additional internal cable wire fixation will increase the stability (Fig. 8.5).

8.3.4 Femoral Shaft Fractures

Intramedullary nail systems (reamed and unreamed nails with their individual pros and cons) are the treatment of choice for femoral shaft fractures. Studies show that the incidence of pulmonary complications is not primarily dependent on the type of stabilization, but is mainly caused by the extent of lung injuries [16]. Several prospective randomized studies comparing reamed and unreamed nails do not show differences in the rate of ARDS, pulmonary complications, and survival rate [17]. Primary intramedullary nailing is contraindicated in grade III open fractures. External fixation is the best method of stabilization in these cases [18] (Fig. 8.6).

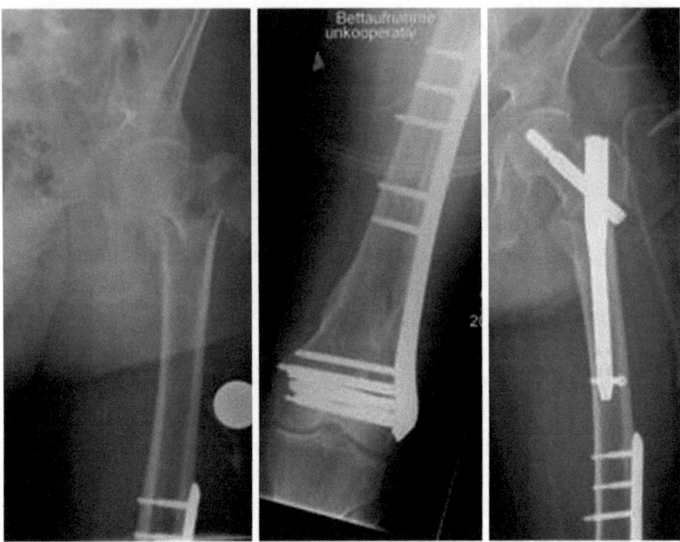

Fig. 8.5 Intertrochanteric femur fracture (A3.2). Closed reduction and internal cephalomedullary nail fixation. A short nail is used because of previous plate fixation of a distal femur fracture

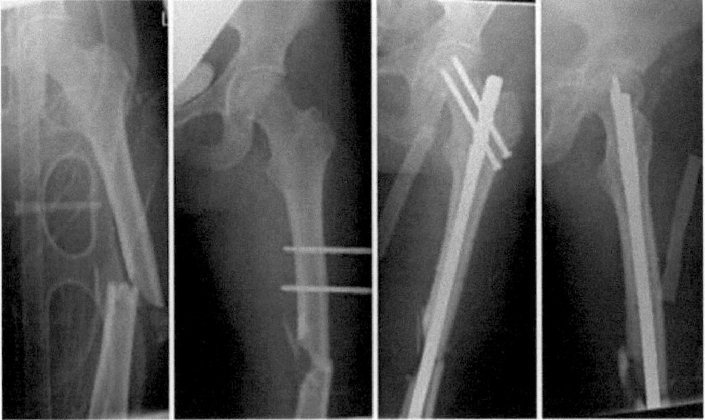

Fig. 8.6 II° open fracture of the femur shaft (B2) in polytraumatized 19-year-old women. Primary closed reduction and external fixation. Secondary nail fixation

8.3.5 *Distal Femoral Fractures*

In hemodynamically unstable patients or higher degrees of soft tissue injuries, a bridging external fixator is a suitable tool for temporary primary stabilization.

Metaphyseal fractures (A2, 3) are the domain of intramedullary nailing (orthograde, retrograde). For B-type fractures compression screw osteosynthesis is recommended.

(Minimally invasive) fixation with locking plates (LISS) is used for comminuted C-type injuries. These fractures are stabilized as follows: stabilization of the joint block by K-wires and/or screws, followed by fixation of the joint block to the shaft by locking compression plates.

8.3.6 *Proximal Tibial Fractures*

Undisplaced extraarticular fractures without soft tissue problems and no risk of a compartment syndrome may be primarily immobilized in a long leg cast.

However, operative treatment with early mobilization is the gold standard.

Displaced avulsions of the intercondylar eminentia (41A1) are fixed by transosseous cable wire or by compression screws. Locking compression plates or plateau buttress plates are used for internal fixation of metaphyseal A2 and A3 fractures. Type B injuries are usually stabilized with compression screws. Large fragments should be stabilized by plates to prevent rotational instability. Articular surface have to be realigned, depressions reduced, and the cancellous bone defects should be filled with autologous bone or bone substitutes. C-type fractures should be treated by plate systems (possibly if needed with additional compression screws). The temporary stabilization by bridging external fixator may be required in cases of critical soft tissue condition, open fractures, vascular injuries, and compartment syndrome, with

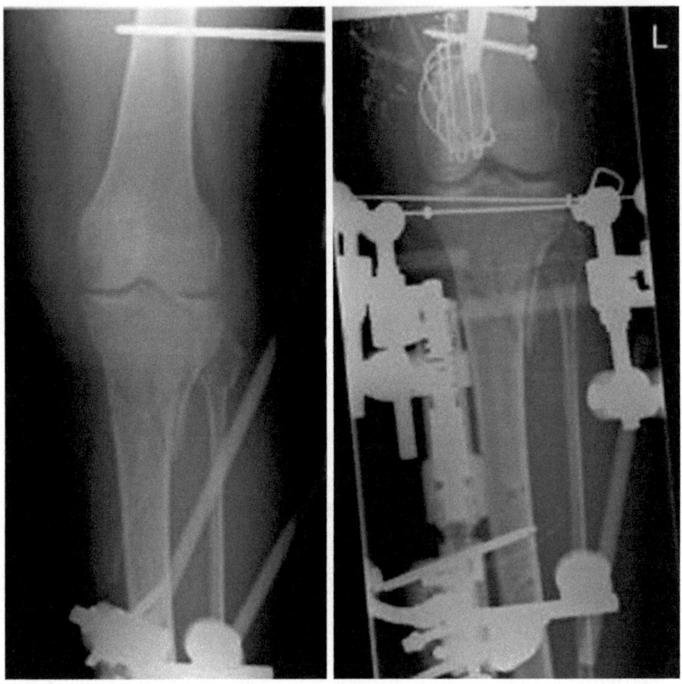

Fig. 8.7 Chain injury with femoral shaft, patella, and proximal tibial fracture. Primary spanning fixator stabilization. Definitive femur care by rodding. Tibial reduction with hybrid fixator (conversed)

secondary definite reconstruction (ORIF or hybrid frame) (Fig. 8.7).

8.3.7 Tibial Shaft Fractures

Analogous to other long bones (femur, humerus) intramedullary nailing is the treatment of choice. The question of reaming or not reaming is answered controversially. The results of a

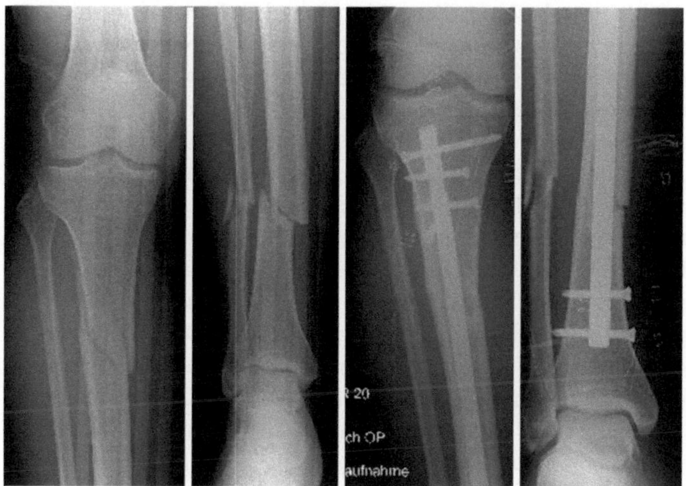

Fig. 8.8 2-level fracture of the tibia. Closed reduction and intramedullary nail fixation

meta-analysis indicate that unreamed intramedullary nails reduce the risk of reoperation, nonunion, and superficial infection compared to external fixator [19]. Compared to unreamed nails, the intramedullary rodding of closed tibial shaft fractures by reamed nails shows a lower rate of pseudarthroses [20]. In comminuted diaphyseal fractures, locking compression plate fixation is an alternative (minimally invasive technique). External fixation is used in critical soft tissue conditions, open fractures, and compartment syndromes (Fig. 8.8).

8.3.8 Distal Tibial Fractures

Intramedullary nailing is possible in distal metaphyseal tibial fractures only if the joint block is large enough for double interlocking. Whenever initial soft tissue conditions prohibit ORIF, temporary external fixator stabilization may be performed. Primary external hybrid fixation is technically demanding. The tibial plafond (pilon tibial) fracture is a comminuted fracture of the distal tibia involving the ankle joint. An axial trauma leads to the epiphyseal and metaphyseal destruction with massive soft tissue problems. In these cases restoration of length and rotation of the lower leg is an option by fixating the fibula (intramedullary wire, plating). An initial joint-bridging external fixator may be necessary for soft tissue protection (optional shortening of tibial length in order to decompress soft tissue), followed by definite internal locking plate fixation (MIPPO technique) after soft tissue recovery. In case of minor soft tissue damage, the pilon can be reconstructed by minimal invasive techniques (K-wire, screw) in the same session.

8.3.9 *Ankle Joint (Malleolar) Fractures*

The descriptive Danis and Weber classification of the distal fibula is based on the localization of the fracture line in relation to the syndesmosis. The Lauge/Hansen classification considers the position of the joint and the direction of the applied force at the moment of the trauma and thus allows a precise assessment of the stability of the ankle joint [21].

Initial external transfixation is indicated in polytraumatized patients with an ISS > 25 and/or a chest trauma of AIS > 3 [22].

For definitive internal fixation one-third tubular plating may be used for the fibula, with and without interfragmentary compression screws.

If there is a rupture of the syndesmosis, the tibiofibular joint must be reduced and temporarily (6 weeks) stabilized with a syndesmotic screw. Open reduction and cancellous screw fixation may be used for the medial malleolus. Comminuted fractures may be fixed by tension band wiring. Fractures of the

Volkmann triangle with a minimum size of 1/5 of the joint surface are stabilized with cannulated screws.

8.3.10 Talus Fractures

Fractures of the talus are caused by axial forces with additional ankle dorsiflexion. Three-fifths of the talar surface is covered with cartilage. Higher-degree fracture dislocations are strongly linked with a compromised blood supply resulting in a high risk of secondary AVN (talus necrosis) with secondary osteoarthritis. Displaced fractures therefore represent an emergency. The classification by Marti/Weber differentiates central and peripheral fractures. Neck fractures are classified according to Hawkins [23]. The procedure of choice is the cannulated screw fixation via the anteromedial approach. Medial ankle osteotomy is required in case of talar fracture dislocation. Weight bearing must be avoided for 10–12 weeks.

8.3.11 Calcaneal Fractures

The fate of this fracture decides itself in the moment of the accident. The classification is according to Essex-Lopresti. Extraarticular fractures of the tuber calcanei (duckbill fracture) can be fixed by minimally invasive cancellous cannulated screws. Intraarticular fractures (joint depression, tongue type, comminuted) require open anatomical reduction via a standard lateral approach. For the anatomical reconstruction of the Böhler angle and the subtalar plane, the Westhues maneuver is helpful. Cancellous bone defects (subtalar voids after reduction of the compressed cancellous bone) must be filled with autologous bone or bone substitutes. The locking compression plate is the implant of choice. No weight bearing for 10–12 weeks. Complications include wound healing disorders, infections, and secondary subtalar arthosis/ankylosis.

References

1. Bardenheuer M, Obertacke U, Waydhas C, Nast-Kolb D et al (2000) Epidemiologie des Schwerverletzten - Eine prospektive Erfassung der präklinischen und klinischen Versorgung. Unfallchirurg 103:355–363
2. Harwood P, Giannoudis P, Van Griensven N et al (2005) Alterations in the systemic inflammatory response after early total care and damage control procedures for femoral shaft fractures in severely injured patients. J Trauma 58:446–452
3. Sturm JA, Oestern HJ, Nerlich ML, Lobenhoffer P (1984) Die primäre Oberschenkelosteosynthese beim Polytrauma: Gefahr oder Gewinn für den Patienten? Langenbecks Arch Chir 364:325–327
4. Wenzel MW (2010) Moderne Osteosynthesetechniken. Extremitätenverletzungen im Rahmen des Polytraumas. Trauma Berufskrankh 12(Suppl 2):160–167
5. Gumina S, Posacchini F (1997) Anterior dislocation of the shoulder in elderly patients. J Bone Joint Surg 79B(4):540–543
6. Neer C (1970) Displaced proximal humerus fractures. Part I. Classification and evaluation. J Bone Joint Surg 52-A:1077–1089
7. Gambirasio R, Riand N, Stern R et al (2001) Total elbow replacement for complex fractures of the distal humerus. An option for the elderly patient. J Bone Joint Surg Br 83(7):974–978
8. Korner J, Lill H, Muller LP (2003) The LCP-concept in the operative treatment of distal humerus fractures – biological, biomechanical and surgical aspects. Injury 34(suppl 02):B20–B30
9. Schatzker J (1987) Olecranon fractures. In: Schatzker J, Tile M (eds) The rationale of operative fracture care. Springer, Berlin/Heidelberg/New York, pp 80–87
10. Metaizeau JP, Lascombes P, Lemelle JL et al (1993) Reduction and fixation of displaced radial neck fractures by closed intramedullary pinning. J Pediatr Orthop 13:355–360
11. Thompson JE (1918) Anatomical methods of approach in operations on the long bones of the Extremities. Ann Surg 68(3):309–329
12. Henry AK (1970) Extensile exposure, 2nd edn. Williams & Wilkins, Baltimore, p 100
13. Essex-Lopresti P (1951) Fractures of the radial head with distal radio-ulnar dislocation: report of two cases. J Bone Joint Surg 33:244–247
14. Pipkin G (1957) Treatment of grade IV fracture-dislocation of the hip. J Bone Joint Surg Am 39:1027–1042

15. Calder SJ, Anderson GH, Jagger C (1996) Unipolar or bipolar prosthesis for displaced intracapsular hip fracture in octogenarians: a randomised prospective study. J Bone Joint Surg Br 78:391–394
16. Bone LB, Babikian G, Stegemann PM (1995) Femoral canal reaming in the polytrauma patient with chest injury: a clinical perspective. Clin Orthop 318:91–94
17. Bosse MJ, Machenzie EJ, Riemer BL, Brumback RJ, McCarthy ML, Burgess AR (1997) Adult respiratory distress syndrome, pneumonia and mortality following thoracic injury and femoral fracture treated either with intramedullary nailing with reaming or with a plate. A comparative study. J Bone Joint Surg Am 79:799–809
18. Scalea TM, Boswell SA, Scott JD, Mitchell KA, Kramer ME, Pollak AN (2000) External fixation as a bridge to intramedullary nailing for patients with multiple injuries and with femur fractures: damage control orthopedics. J Trauma 48:613–623
19. Bhandari M, Guyatt GH, Swiontkowski MF, Schemitsch EH (2001) Treatment of open fractures of the shaft of the tibia. J Bone Joint Surg Br 83:62–68
20. Larsen LB, Madsen JE, Hoiness PR, Ovre S (2004) Should insertion of intramedullary nails for tibial fractures be with or without reaming? A prospective, randomized study with 3.8 years' follow up. J Orthop Trauma 18:144–149
21. Lauge-Hansen N (1950) Fractures of the ankle. II. Combined experimental-surgical and experimental-roentgenologic investigations. Arch Surg 60:947–985
22. Ankin N (1998) Surgical treatment of fractures of long bones in a patient with multiple injuries. Klin Khir 7:41–44
23. Hawkins LG (1970) Fractures of the neck of the talus. J Bone Joint Surg Am 52:991

Chapter 9
Minimally Invasive Approach and Endovascular Techniques for Vascular Trauma

Joseph J. DuBose, Megan Brenner, and Thomas M. Scalea

The recent emergence of endovascular technologies has expanded the modalities available for use in the treatment of vascular injury. Initially employed in the treatment of atherosclerotic vascular disease, endovascular modalities have increasingly been utilized for specific vascular trauma indications. The position of endovascular approaches in algorithms for vascular injury treatment, however, continues to evolve. To date, these tools have most commonly been employed at challenging vascular injury locations or for those injuries traditionally associated with poor outcomes when approached via open modalities. This chapter will outline the published results from these

Electronic supplementary material is available in the online version of this chapter at (doi:10.1007/978-88-470-5403-5_9).

J.J. DuBose, MD, FACS • M. Brenner, MD, MS, FACS
T.M. Scalea, MD, FACS (✉)
Department of Surgery, R Adams Cowley
Shock Trauma Center, University of Maryland
Medical System, 22 South Greene Street,
T3R35, Baltimore, MD 21201, USA
e-mail: jjd3c@yahoo.com; mbrenner@umm.edu; tscalea@umm.edu

S. Di Saverio et al. (eds.), *Trauma Surgery*,
DOI 10.1007/978-88-470-5403-5_9, © Springer-Verlag Italia 2014

experiences. We will also discuss the potential for future applications of endovascular treatment as well as the present challenges to increased utilization of these technologies.

9.1 Endovascular Experience with Management of Thoracic Aortic Injuries

Thoracic endovascular aortic repair (TEVAR) has, in recent years, emerged as the standard of care for a significant portion of traumatic aortic injuries that were traditionally treated by open surgical means [1–5]. The largest examinations on the topic were conducted by the Demetriades and colleagues of the American Association for the Surgery of Trauma (AAST) Thoracic Aortic Injury Study Group in a large prospective observational trial of blunt thoracic aortic injuries [6, 7]. In the first of these reports, the investigators noted that 65 % of the 193 patients with thoracic aortic injury (TAI) underwent endovascular stent graft repair (TEVAR), with the remaining patients undergoing open repair. After risk adjustment for mortality, the researchers noted that the TEVAR group required significantly fewer blood transfusions and had a significantly lower mortality than open surgical counterparts (adjusted odds ratio 8.42; 95 % CI [2.76–25.69]; adjusted p value <0.001). They did, however, note that 20 % of TEVAR patients developed some form of device-related complications but that a lower rate of these complications occurred in centers with higher volumes of TEVAR utilization.

The same group of researchers also reported on the trends in utilization of TEVAR between two phases of study separated by a decade (AAST1, completed in 1997 and spanning 30 months vs. AAST2, completed in 2007 and lasting 26 months). The group noted a profound trend in the utilization of TEVAR when comparing these two periods. During the period of AAST1, all TAI were repaired utilizing open means. In contrast, by the time of the 2007 study conclusion, only 35.2 % were managed with open surgical intervention – the remaining undergoing TEVAR. The authors also noted both a significant decrease in TAI-associated mortality (22 % vs. 13 %, $p=0.02$) and incidence of procedure-related paraplegia (8.7 % vs. 1.6 %, $p=0.001$) over time.

Despite the emergence of TEVAR, several key elements of endovascular treatment of thoracic aortic injury require additional examination. Initially utilized devices were often improvised or were designed for the treatment of abdominal aneurysmal disease. Many subsequent complications in stent deployment were, accordingly, related to issues in failure of the device to adequately conform safely to the contour of the thoracic aorta. Additionally, the diagnosis and treatment of inadvertent or intentional coverage of the subclavian or other arch vessels was poorly understood. Although the evolution in endovascular technologies and improved management algorithms has mitigated much of these risks, further research is required. In particular, long-term follow-up of these devices is required. Given the relative younger age of many trauma patients and associated smaller diameter of the thoracic aorta, the potential for stent malfunction, migration, or other complications over time has not been well documented.

9.2   Endovascular Experience with Management of Cerebrovascular Injuries

The treatment and outcome of cerebrovascular injuries is influenced by many factors, including the mechanism, type of injury, and associated neurologic function. These injuries may be associated with considerable mortality and high rates of neurologic impairment. Several types of injuries may result from cerebrovascular trauma, regardless of mechanism. Those that do not commonly result in the operative indications of hemorrhage or expanding hematoma include intimal flaps, dissections, and pseudoaneurysms. The natural history and appropriate management of these injuries remain ill defined. Anticoagulation following blunt carotid injury is known to be associated with improved outcome following blunt trauma, but some types of injuries are more likely to fail conservative therapy. It has been reported that up to 40 % of patients in the modern era may require endovascular intervention for these injuries [9].

Borrowing on the expanding experience with the use of endovascular stents for cerebrovascular disease, carotid stenting has been utilized for high extracranial internal carotid lesions. These types of interventions are ideally suited for this region, where surgical approaches are most difficult, and are associated with a high rate of local and cerebrovascular complications. An endovascular approach may also prove particularly useful in the treatment of select type of internal carotid injuries, as surgical resection or repair of internal carotid pseudoaneurysms in particular is associated with a high mortality rate and high incidence of cerebral complications.

In the largest review on this topic to date, DuBose and colleagues [10] identified experiences from 113 patients undergoing carotid stenting that were reported in the literature from 1994 to 2008. The injury types treated by stenting included pseudoaneurysm (60.2 %), arteriovenous fistula (16.8 %) dissection (14.2 %), partial transection (4.4 %), occlusion (2.7 %), intimal flap (0.9 %), and aneurysm (0.9 %). Over radiographic and clinical follow-up periods ranging from 2 weeks to 2 years, a follow-up patency of 79.6 % was documented. New neurologic deficits after stent placement occurred in only 3.5 % of patients, improved over historical experiences with open repair after trauma. Although these initial experiences are promising, no large prospective study on this topic has yet been conducted, and further research is warranted.

9.3 Endovascular Experience with Management of Axillo-subclavian Injuries

Injuries to the subclavian and axillary arteries continue to be associated with high rates of morbidity and mortality. In one of the landmark series on these injuries, Demetriades and colleagues at Los Angeles County + University of Southern California Hospital [8] examined penetrating subclavian and axillary injuries, identifying 79 patients with these injuries over approximately 4 years. The associated overall mortality was 34.2 %. Even after excluding those patients in extremis requiring resuscitative thoracotomies, mortality remained considerable at 14.8 %. These experiences, combined with the confined anatomical relationships of the thoracic inlet, contribute to the complexity attributed to open surgical treatment of subclavian/ axillary trauma. These challenges have made injuries at this location an attractive target for study of the utilization of endovascular technologies.

In the largest review of this topic, conducted by DuBose et al. [11], investigators identified 32 published reports of endovascular treatment of subclavian or axillary artery injuries with sufficient information for review. These reports described 160 patients (150 subclavian; 10 axillary), the majority of which (56.3 %) were due to penetrating injuries. Lesions treated included pseudoaneurysm, arteriovenous fistula, perforation, occlusion, partial or complete transection, and dissection. Only six procedure-related complications were reported. The only reported periprocedural mortality reported was a death occurring in the angiography suite after successful deployment of an endovascular stent had been completed. Overall, radiographic and clinical follow-up periods ranging from hospital discharge to 70 months were reported, with no device-related infections, migrations, or acute limb-threatening ischemic events reported among the 160 reported cases. The authors documented an asymptomatic patency rate of 84.4 % for the duration of available follow-up. This group concluded that, despite uncertainties in patient selection and optimal management algorithms, early results of endovascular treatment for properly selected subclavian and axillary injuries are promising.

9.4 Endovascular Experience with Management of Vascular Injury at Other Locations

Endovascular management of vascular injury at other anatomical locations has also been proposed [12, 13]. Treatment of visceral [14], iliac [15], and even peripheral artery injuries [16, 17] has been described. To date, however, there have been no large prospective studies in these settings, and availability of data is limited to case reports or small case series. Defining the optimal utilization of endovascular therapy for injuries at more anatomically accessible sites will require additional study.

9.5 Endovascular Vascular Control as an Adjunct to Open Surgical Intervention

As the exploration of endovascular application for trauma has continued to evolve, so too has the potential application of this technology. Many early studies have focused on direct comparisons of open versus endovascular interventions. Increasingly, however, awareness that these two approaches may work in compliment with one another has arisen. So-called hybrid approaches may hold considerable promise in the treatment of vascular injury. Endovascular balloons have been effectively utilized for proximal occlusion, dilation, and stent deployment in the treatment of atherosclerotic disease. Increasingly, their use in hybrid vascular trauma applications has also been examined.

The use of endovascular occlusion for trauma indications is not an entirely new concept. Scalea and Sclafani from Kings County Hospital of Brooklyn, New York, first described this technique in 1991 [18]. In recent years, however, several groups of investigators have subjected the utilization of this practice to greater scrutiny using animal models [19–21]. Early results suggest that the application of endovascular technologies may provide rapid control of proximal arterial hemorrhage, facilitating a more controlled effort at exposure and operative repair. Future study on these types of hybrid approaches is likely to demonstrate the complementary nature of endovascular and open surgical interventions for vascular trauma.

9.6   Potential Complications and Present Limitations of Endovascular Management

Despite recent advances of endovascular trauma applications, it is paramount that trauma providers understand the specific complications unique to these technologies. These begin with the skill sets required to adequately utilize these innovations. At present the techniques and tools of endovascular intervention largely belong to those specialists formally trained in interventional radiology or vascular surgery. As hybrid approaches become more common, however, these conditions may change. Several studies, most notably the aforementioned AAST TEVAR experience, have also demonstrated the relationship between volume of procedures performed and subsequent outcomes. These data suggest that endovascular trauma management is best accomplished at high-volume trauma centers with experienced providers.

Endovascular approaches also have specific potential complications that may require specialist support to manage effectively. This may be particularly true for stent coverage of vascular injuries. Endoleaks, stent migration, and prosthetic failure are all potential management dilemmas that will require capable subspecialty support to effectively treat.

Access site complications may also be common. Many of the present devices utilized for trauma endovascular intervention require fairly sizeable deployment systems for device introduction into peripheral arteries. Particularly for young trauma victims with smaller diameter arteries, these device sizes are presently problematic. Continued evolution of endovascular technologies may someday ameliorate this risk, but, at present, endovascular device companies have been slower to embrace these special concerns for trauma applications.

Perhaps the greatest present limitation of endovascular technologies for trauma is the lack of adequate follow-up data. As the ease of utilization improves, so too must the ability of trauma providers to determine the durability of endovascular intervention for injury. The recently initiated PROspective Observational Vascular Injury Trial (PROOVIT) study of the American Association for the Surgery of Trauma (AAST) is one modality that holds promise in this regard. This study is designed to capture initial endovascular and open vascular injury treatments at a wide variety of anatomical locations – as well as long-term follow-up data. It is the hope of the study group that this information will help to define the optimal utilization of endovascular technologies for trauma.

9.7 Conclusion

The role of endovascular management for vascular injury continues to evolve. These technologies, both in isolation and in hybrid coordination with open surgical intervention, hold considerable promise for the future. Well established already for specific indications, further study is needed to determine the optimal role of endovascular techniques in vascular injury management algorithms.

References

1. Garcia-Toca M, Naugton PA, Matsumura JS, Morasch MD, Kibbe MR, Rodriguez HE, Pearce WH, Eskandari MK (2010) Endovascular repair of blunt traumatic thoracic aortic injuries: seven-year single-center experience. Arch Surg 145(7):679–683
2. Willis M, Neschis D, Menaker J, Lilly M, Scalea T (2011) Stent grafting for a distal thoracic aortic injury. Vasc Endovascular Surg 45(2): 187–190
3. Neschis DG, Moainie S, Flinn WR, Scalea TM, Bartlett ST, Griffith BP (2009) Endograft repair of traumatic aortic injury-a technique in evolution: a single institution's experience. Ann Surg 250(3):377–382
4. Neschis DG, Scalea TM (2010) Endovascular repair of traumatic aortic injuries. Adv Surg 44:281–292
5. Demetriades D, Velmahos GC, Scalea TM, Jurkovich GJ, Karmy-Jones R, Teixeira PG, Hemmila MR, O'Connor JV, McKenney MO, Moore FO, London J, Singh MJ, Spaniolas K, Keel M, Sugrue M, Wahl WL, Hill J, Wall MJ, Moore EE, Lineen E, Marguiles D, Malka V, Chan LS (2009) Blunt traumatic thoracic aortic injuries: early or delayed repair—results of an American Association for the Surgery of Trauma prospective study. J Trauma 66(4):967–973
6. Demetriades D, Velmahos GC, Scalea TM, Jurkovich GJ, Karmy-Jones R, Teixeira PG, Hemmila MR, O'Connor JV, McKenney MO, Moore FO, London J, Singh MJ, Spaniolas K, Keel M, Sugrue M, Wahl WL, Hill J, Wall MJ, Moore EE, Lineen E, Marguiles D, Malka V, Chan LS, American Association for the Surgery of Trauma Thoracic Aortic Injury Study Group (2008) Operative repair or endovascular stent graft in blunt traumatic thoracic aortic injuries: results of an American Association for the Surgery of Trauma Multicenter Study. J Trauma 64(3):561–570; discussion 570–571
7. Demetriades D, Velmahos GC, Scalea TM, Jurkovich GJ, Karmy-Jones R, Teixeira PG, Hemmila MR, O'Connor JV, McKenney MO, Moore FO, London J, Singh MJ, Spaniolas K, Keel M, Sugrue M, Wahl WL,

Hill J, Wall MJ, Moore EE, Lineen E, Marguiles D, Malka V, Chan LS (2008) Diagnosis and treatment of blunt thoracic aortic injuries: changing perspectives. J Trauma 64(6):1415–1418; discussion 1418–1419

8. Demtriades D, Chahwan S, Gomez H, Peng R, Velmahos G, Murray J, Asensio J, Bongard F (1999) Penetrating injuries to the subclavian and axillary vessels. J Am Coll Surg 188(3):290–295

9. DiCocco JM, Fabian TC, Emmett KP, Magnotti LJ, Zarzaur BL, Bate BG, Muhlbauer MS, Khan N, Kelly JM, Williams JS, Croce MA (2011) Optimal outcomes for patients with blunt cerebrovascular injury (BCVI): tailoring treatment to the lesion. J Am Coll Surg 212(4):549–557; discussion 557–559

10. DuBose J, Recinos G, Teixeira PG, Inaba K, Demetriades D (2008) Endovascular stenting for the treatment of traumatic internal carotid injuries: expanding experience. J Trauma 65(6):1561–1566

11. DuBose JJ, Rajani R, Gilani R, Arthurs ZA, Morrison JJ, Clouse WD, Rasmussen TE, For the Endovascular Skills for Trauma and Resuscitative Surgery (ESTARS) Working Group (2012) Endovascular management of axillo-subclavian arterial injury: a review of published experience. Injury 43(11):1785–1792

12. White R, Krajcer Z, Johnson M, Williams D, Bacharach M, O'Malley E (2006) Results of a multicenter trial for the treatment of traumatic vascular injury with a covered stent. J Trauma 60(6):1189–1195; discussion 1195–1196

13. Starnes BW, Arthurs ZM (2006) Endovascular management of vascular trauma. Perspect Vasc Surg Endovasc Ther 18(2):114–129

14. Boufi M, Bordon S, Dona B, Hartung O, Sarran A, Nadeau S, Maurin C, Alimi YS (2011) Unstable patients with retroperitoneal vascular trauma: an endovascular approach. Ann Vasc Surg 25(3):352–358

15. Anderson CA, Strumpf RK, Diethrich EB (2008) Endovascular management of a large post-traumatic iliac arteriovenous fistula: utilization of a septal occlusion device. J Vasc Surg 48(6):1597–1599

16. Piffaretti G, Tozzi M, Lomazzi C, Rivolta N, Caronno R, Lagana D, Carrafiello G, Castelli P (2007) Endovascular treatment for traumatic injuries of the peripheral arteries following blunt trauma. Injury 38(9):1091–1097

17. Trellopoulos G, Georgiadis GS, Asianidou EA, Nikolopoulos ES, Pitta X, Papachristodoulou A, Lazarides MK (2012) Endovascular management of peripheral artery trauma in patients presenting in hemorrhagic shock. J Cardiovasc Surg (Torino) 53(4):495–506

18. Scalea TM, Sclafani SJ (1991) Angiographically placed balloons for arterial control: a description of technique. J Trauma 31(12):1671–1677

19. Morrison JJ, Percival TJ, Markov NP, Villamaria C, Scott DJ, Saches KA, Spencer JR, Rasmussen TE (2012) Aortic balloon occlusion is effective in controlling pelvic hemorrhage. J Surg Res 177(2):341–347
20. Stannard A, Eliason JL, Rasmussen TE (2011) Resuscitative endovascular balloon occlusion of the aorta (REBOA) as an adjunct for hemorrhagic shock. J Trauma 71(6):1869–1872
21. White JM, Cannon JW, Stannard A, Markov NP, Spencer JR, Rasmussen TE (2011) Endovascular balloon occlusion of the aorta is superior to resuscitative thoracotomy with aortic clamping in a porcine model of hemorrhagic shock. Surgery 150(3):400–409

Chapter 10
Interventional Techniques for Hemorrhage Control in Trauma

Robert Short, Alan Murdock, Phillip Orons, and Andrew B. Peitzman

Interventional radiologic techniques have become a mainstay in the management of trauma ranging from hemorrhage control (i.e., endovascular balloon occlusion, stenting, and embolization) to the management of complications (i.e., drainage of abscesses and placement of inferior vena caval filters). This chapter will provide a broad overview of the diagnostic assessment, equipment, techniques, and their specific applications in the care of the injured patient as it relates to solid organ injury, pelvic bleeding, and resuscitation assisted by aortic balloon occlusion. Endovascular techniques specifically applicable for great vessel injury will be covered elsewhere in this handbook.

R. Short, MD, PhD • P. Orons, MD
Division of General Surgery, Department of Radiology,
University of Pittsburgh Physicians, Pittsburgh,
PA 15213, USA

A. Murdock, Col, USAF, MC • A.B. Peitzman, MD (✉)
Division of General Surgery, Department of Surgery,
University of Pittsburgh Physicians, Pittsburgh,
PA 15213, USA
e-mail: peitzmanab@upmc.edu

S. Di Saverio et al. (eds.), *Trauma Surgery*,
DOI 10.1007/978-88-470-5403-5_10, © Springer-Verlag Italia 2014

10.1 Diagnostic Radiologic Assessment

10.1.1 Computed Tomography

Computed tomography (CT) is the principal diagnostic test in hemodynamically stable trauma patients due to its widespread availability, speed, and unambiguous anatomic detail. With the advent of multislice CT scanners, bleeding and vascular injuries have become more readily identified. In addition, CT scanners with 16 slices and above are able to provide rapid angiographic evaluation of any vascular region. Computed tomography angiography (CTA) is the primary assessment modality in trauma for suspected vascular injury. Keys to success in performing CTA include (1) contrast timing – bolus must be timed to achieve peak arterial enhancement of the main regions of interest, (2) table timing – table movement can move faster than contrast bolus; therefore acquisition rate may need to be adjusted for some patients, and (3) multiplanar reformatting, a technique which assembles cross-sectional images into an image more consistent with conventional angiography. Most CT scanners today have preprogrammed reconstruction algorithms optimizing the imaging quality of the various CTA scenarios. Typical CTA protocols require IV administration of contrast of around 100 ml. While CTA often can localize bleeding, intervention must be carried out surgically or in the angiography suite (Fig. 10.1).

10.1.2 Angiography

The majority of angiography is currently performed using digital subtraction. Digital subtraction angiography (DSA) provides visualization of blood vessels by subtracting out background structures before contrast injection. DSA can be performed with multi-station or stepping table (bolus chase) techniques. Multi-station DSA is performed in sections, each with its own injection (e.g., upper arm, lower arm, hand). This usually gives the

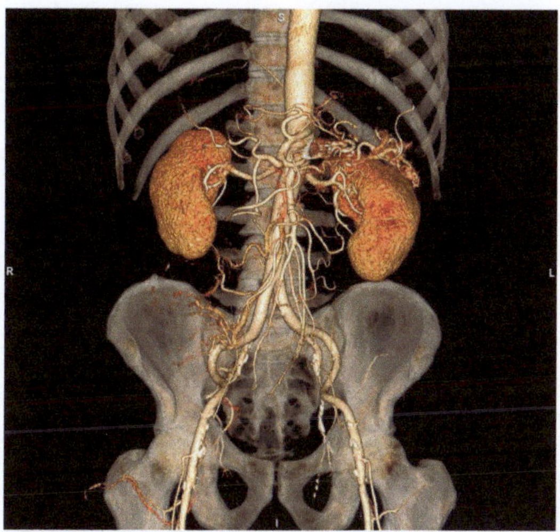

Fig. 10.1 A 3-D reconstruction from CT angiogram of the abdomen and pelvis

best images particularly for peripheral angiography but increases radiation dose and contrast administration. Stepping table DSA is used only in peripheral angiography. The C-arm or table moves in a series of overlapping steps with a single bolus of contrast injection. This technique usually requires a more experienced technician and is of limited utility except in bilateral lower extremity pathology (Fig. 10.2).

10.2 Equipment

10.2.1 Fluoroscopy

Most modern angiography units use pulsed fluoroscopy where radiation is produced in a pulsating fashion instead of a continuous beam. The pulses typically range from 2 to 30 pulses per second. The primary advantage of pulsed fluoroscopy is a

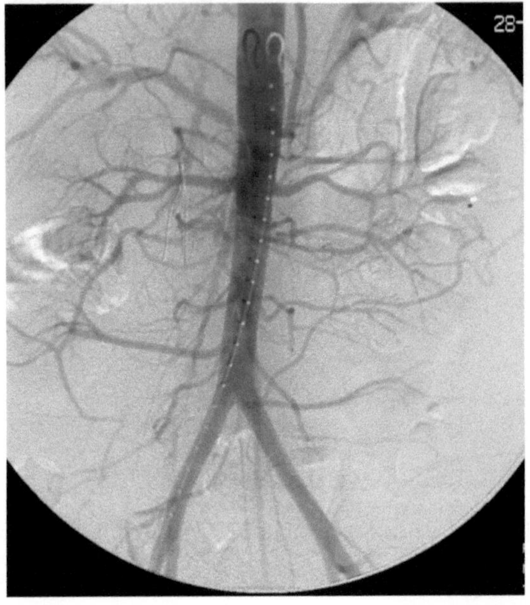

Fig. 10.2 Digital subtraction angiography (DSA) of the abdomen and pelvis (AP view)

significant reduction in radiation dose. The goal of fluoroscopy is to hold the radiation exposure to both patient and operator to a minimum while still providing the image detail necessary for the given situation. In addition to the use of pulsed fluoroscopy, this can be achieved by keeping the image intensifier or flat-panel detector close to the patient, centering over the region of interest, judicious use of collimation, moving the table before screening when changing positions, and optimizing single angiographic runs to sort out anatomy. Judicious application of fluoroscopy and features such as "last image hold" where the last image is displayed on the monitor also help reduce radiation exposure to the patient, technologists, nurses, and physicians.

10.2.2   Power Injectors

Power injectors deliver a controlled bolus of contrast. They have significant advantages over hand injections by delivering contrast boluses with higher flow rates, consistent volumes, and precise timing. Parameters settings include flow rate (ml/s), total volume (ml), pressure rate rise, linear rise, maximum pressure (psi), and injection delay. Flow rate is selected on the basis of vessel diameter and blood flow. Volume depends on the desired column length and size of area of interest. Pressure rate rise is the time to peak pressure and typically set at 0.4 s. Although most modern angiographic catheters have very high pressure tolerance, catheter-specific maximum pressure is set to avoid any chance of catheter rupture. The pressure generated by a power contrast injection is dependent on contrast viscosity, flow rate, catheter luminal diameter, and catheter material and length. Linear rise is the time required to reach the maximum flow rate. It is used to avoid catheter recoil and potential vessel injury. Rise time depends on catheter size and position. For example, a linear rise of 0.2 s is typical for multi-side hole catheters but a longer time (0.4–0.8 s) may be required for an end-hole catheter. Injection delay can be variable depending on the distance of the area of interest from the catheter delivering the contrast bolus.

10.2.3   Vascular Access Sheaths

When bleeding is suspected, vascular access must be gained by an artery. Typically this is the femoral artery, although brachial or even radial arterial access methods have been employed. Vascular sheaths provide an atraumatic conduit for vascular access and are particularly helpful when multiple catheter exchanges are required. By convention, a sheath size is rated for size of the catheter it will accept in its lumen but has a larger outside diameter. For example, a 5 Fr sheath will accept a 5 Fr catheter (1 "French" equals approximately 0.33 mm) but produces a 6.5 Fr hole in the artery. The sheath has a hemostatic valve where catheters are inserted and a sidearm for flushing to which a "flush bag" can be attached to prevent thrombus formation at the tip of the sheath.

10.2.4　Guidewires

Guidewires serve to negotiate a pathway from entry access to target area. Along with the choice of an appropriate catheter, the guidewire used is the key element in the success of any selective or superselective catheterization and ultimately the success or failure of any diagnostic or interventional procedure. Guidewires are divided into two major categories: non-steerable and steerable. Non-steerable guidewires provide a rail for catheters to be advanced into crude position but not navigate into select branch vessels. Typical examples of non-steerable guidewires include the following: J guidewire (most common), Straight, Bentson, Rosen, Amplatz, and Lunderquist. Steerable guidewires have shaped or shapeable angled tips allowing them to be selectively rotated and directed through tight stenoses or areas of tortuosity into branch vessels.

Selection of guidewire application is further based on diameter, length, material (e.g., stainless steel or nitinol), lubricity (hydrophilic or not), wire tip shape, and overall stiffness. Most guidewires are either microwires (0.010–0.018 in.) or standard (0.025–0.038 in.). The majority of cases start with use of a standard 0.035 in. guidewire which will fit through 4 or 5 Fr catheter. Small caliber wires (typically 0.010–0.018 in.) are used with microcatheters, usually coaxially through a 5 Fr base catheter. Length of the guidewire is critical when considering catheter exchanges to gain favorable position. A standard guidewire is

145–180 cm, but longer wires may be required for working from groin to upper limb or visceral circulation. Wire tips are floppy and atraumatic at one end and rigid at the other end. The length of the floppy tip can vary and application is based on optimizing the transition zone (floppy to stiff portion) within the target vessel. Wire stiffness is a key criterion in selection of non-steerable wires. Stiffness choice is made based on task required. For example, a 5 Fr diagnostic catheter can be advanced over a standard guidewire, but, depending on body habitus or vascular tortuosity, a large sheath or guiding catheter used to deliver a stent may require the use of a stiffer guidewire. Very flexible microwires with shapeable tips are often required to select small vessels, over which a microcatheter can be positioned for superselective embolization.

10.2.5   Catheters

Like guidewires, catheters are divided into two categories: nonselective (diagnostic) and selective. Catheters are named for their outer lumen size (e.g., 5 French). Nonselective catheters, also known as flush catheters, are used to inject medium to large-sized vessels and have multiple side holes to deliver large boluses of contrast. A pigtail catheter is the most commonly used nonselective catheter. Pigtail catheters are marketed in a variety of iterations and have both end and side holes which provide largest flow at the end with homogenous contrast bolus from the side holes. Maximum flow rate of catheters depend on luminal diameter, length, and number of side holes. The maximum injection rate and injection pressure is listed packaging and catheter hub.

Selective catheters have a wide variety of shapes and are used to selectively access branch vessels. Selective catheters may have end hole only or end and side holes. End-hole catheters should not be used indiscriminately with power injectors due to

Table 10.1 Measurement standard nomenclature for angiography catheters, wires, and sheaths

French sizes (circumference mm)	Inches	Centimeters
Angiographic catheter (outer)	Wire diameter	Wire length
Guide-catheter size (outer)	Catheter lumen	Catheter length
Sheath size (inner)		Sheath length

the high flow jet created which may lead to possible vessel injury or dissection. Catheters are further classified by their material (e.g., hydrophilic) and their composition, braided or non-braided. A braided catheter has a small amount of metallic fiber woven into the walls which makes the catheter more steerable and improves trackability.

Common selective catheters include Cobra, Berenstein, Sidewinder, and Headhunter. Each of these catheters is designed for specific target regions such as head and neck, aortic arch, visceral, and peripheral. Most cases start with a diagnostic catheter (e.g., 5 Fr pigtail), and then selective catheters are chosen based on the intended treatment vessel, but changes are often made during a case based on the given anatomy. A microcatheter is employed coaxially for more distal access into smaller vessels where advancing larger catheters might be difficult or impossible, might be occlusive, or cause vessel spasm or injury (Table 10.1).

10.3 Interventional Technique

It must be noted that while techniques for access, vascular catheterization, and endovascular treatment are described in this chapter, these types of interventions should not be performed without first having received direct training and guidance by an experienced endovascular interventionalist.

10.3.1   Vascular Access

Access puncture sites are fixed and compressible over bone for hemostasis. The common femoral artery (CFA) is the most widely used site because of the size of the vessel and lowest risk of complications at the site. Brachial access is occasionally employed but even small amount of hemorrhage at this site carries potential adjacent nerve damage. The choice of ipsilateral or contralateral, or antegrade or retrograde femoral access for lower extremity arteriography or intervention depends on the index of suspicion of injury, intended treatment plan, and age and clinical status of the patient. For example, one might not want to access the right common femoral artery in an individual with a right acetabular fracture. The elderly often have markedly tortuous iliac vasculature that might make contralateral catheterization difficult, and marked obesity might make safe antegrade femoral access difficult or impossible.

The CFA courses over the medial half of the femoral head. Pulse is typically used as the landmark, but position of the femoral head should be checked with fluoroscopy as the inguinal crease is not a reliable landmark, particularly in obese patients. Ultrasound-guided puncture can facilitate arterial access in difficult cases or may even be utilized on a routine basis.

It is recommended that puncture of the femoral artery should be at the level of the midpoint of the femoral head. The skin entry site and course of the needle should account for this such that a more inferior skin entry will be required. Puncturing the CFA too high (above the inguinal ligament) increases the risk of bleeding due to inability to compress the artery after sheath removal. Too low of a puncture carries similar risk but may lead to occlusion of the superficial femoral artery. Access of the CFA is typically performed either with a micropuncture set or standard vascular access kit. The micropuncture set uses a smaller gauge needle (21 G) and accepts a 0.018-in. wire with floppy tip. Once the vessel is accessed with the 21 G needle, the 0.018-in. wire is passed, over which a two-part dilator is introduced. The 3 Fr inner component accepts and accommodates the small 0.018 in., and the outer 4 Fr component has a 0.035-in. diameter. Once the inner component is removed, a standard 0.035-in. guidewire can be passed and allow the placement of a vascular sheath. The standard access kit uses an 18/19 G needle that will accept a 0.035-in. guidewire. The micropuncture set has the advantage of securing an optimal puncture with less risk of trauma to the vessel.

10.3.2   Sheath Placement/Passage of Guidewire

Access of the artery with a micropuncture set as described above is recommended. With the 21 G needle in place and pulsatile blood return confirmed, the 0.018-in. wire should be slowly advanced under fluoroscopic guidance. The needle position over the femoral head can be confirmed with the wire in place. If too high or too low, withdraw the needle and wire, apply pressure for several minutes, and try again. When manipulating the wire, the tip of the wire should be in view at all times. If there is any resistance, withdraw a few centimeters, and then advance again looking for deviation from the anticipated path. If the 0.018-in. wire will not advance intraluminally, it is likely the needle tip has been advanced too far into the vessel wall. Withdraw the wire, check for pulsatile flow, and reposition the needle if necessary. If the wire is intraluminal and will not advance, ensure that the wire is taking the anticipated path and not in a branch vessel. If redirection is not successful, a 4 Fr dilator can be inserted to secure the access. Make certain that the dilator can be aspirated. Gently inject contrast to confirm intraluminal position then hand-inject an angiogram to identify the problem. Once access is established with the 4 Fr micropuncture set, the inner portion and 0.018-in. wire are removed and a 0.035-in. guidewire is advanced through the lumen. A J-wire with a very floppy tip (e.g., LLT or Benson) is the most commonly used starter guidewire. Once this wire is in place, typically a 5 Fr 10-cm sheath is placed over the wire. Use of steerable hydrophilic wires or shaped catheters may be necessary to navigate diseased or tortuous vessels. Always ensure a suitable length of the guidewire in the vessel before introducing a sheath/dilator or exchanging a catheter.

10.3.3   Introduction of Catheter

Catheter selection is dependent on the procedure. The catheter should be move easily over a guidewire which must be fixed and under tension (i.e., the system must be kept straightened). Always insert an ample amount of guidewire under fluoroscopic visualization into the vessels before passing the catheter. The wire leads the catheter into a large vessel. The wire is then advanced to the target followed by the catheter placement into the branch vessel for angiography or intervention. Catheter shape, in addition to steerable guidewires, will be the main determinant of the ability to successfully catheterize the intended target vessel. Most microcatheters have radiopaque tips to allow easy identification of the catheter tip. A small hand injection of contrast under fluoroscopy should always be performed to gauge catheter position and blood flow before DSA is performed.

10.3.4   Performing an Angiogram

Three keys elements are involved in performing a high-quality diagnostic angiogram: (1) appropriate placement of the catheter tip, (2) appropriate contrast rate injection and image acquisition rate, and (3) imaging angle. For example, performing an

Table 10.2 Angiography typical standards for aortogram

Aortogram	Position	Contrast (cc/s)	Total (cc)	Frames/s	View
Arch	1 cm distal AV	20	40	4–6	LAO 40°
Abdominal	T12 or L1	15	30	4	LAO 10–15°
Pelvis	1–2 cm prox bifurcation	10	20	2–4	AP, LAO 25°, RAO 25°

LAO left anterior oblique, *AP* anterior posterior, *RAO* right anterior oblique

aortogram can be accomplished at three major levels: arch, abdominal, and pelvis. The catheter for arch aortogram should be in the proximal ascending arch typically by "bouncing" the catheter tip off the aortic value and pulling back 1 cm. Contrast (100 % strength) is then injected at approximately 20 cc for 2 s for a total of 40 cc. Image acquisition is set at 4–6 frames/s with steep left anterior oblique view to evaluate the origins and avoid superimposition of the great vessels. Orthogonal or varying projections are often necessary for complete vascular evaluation. Table 10.2 provides standard injection and acquisition rates for various anatomic locations. Note that these volumes and rates may vary higher or lower depending on patient age, vascular diameter, cardiac output, and blood pressure.

10.4   Trauma Vascular Interventions

Trauma comprises a wide range of injuries from both blunt and penetrating mechanisms. A high index of suspicion, early recognition, and timely intervention are critical in alleviating the deadly triad of coagulopathy, hypothermia, and acidosis. The patient's clinical condition is the most important consideration in deciding between open surgical versus endovascular intervention. It is difficult to perform angiography and resuscitate a multi-injured patient, but imaging-guided endovascular intervention has a key role in addressing a single life-threatening focal bleeding source. Once the decision has been made to proceed with angiography, establish the objectives of the study, and focus on the major targets first.

10.4.1 Diagnosis

Rapid diagnosis of potential trauma hemorrhage via plain radiographs (chest and pelvis radiographs) as well as ultrasound (FAST – focused abdominal sonogram for trauma) is critical in the assessment of hemodynamically unstable patients. However, CT has become the standard in the assessment of the hemodynamically stable patient and most useful in screening for solid organ, mesenteric, pelvic, and retroperitoneal bleeding. Indication for angiography in thoracic and abdominal trauma is now mainly based on active contrast extravasation on CT angiography.

In penetrating trauma, injury is usually identified by contrast extravasation or the presence of pseudoaneurysms. Occasionally, there may be significant adventitial and medial tears without intimal injury leading to an almost normal angiogram. It is important to evaluate for spasm and vascular deviation secondary to hematoma.

The main mechanisms for blunt arterial injury are stretch and compression which may cause shearing of the vessel. All three arterial layers can be injured and lead to the intramural thrombosis. Minor injury may cause arterial spasm, whereas severe injuries often present as dissections of varying degrees which may ultimately result in rupture or occlusion. Evaluation of distal runoff in extremities is essential for surgical planning.

Thoracic aortic injury is a life-threatening injury with most patients dying prior to arrival to a hospital. Aortic injury is caused by a combination of factors. Direct compression of the thorax causes a sudden increase in cardiac output while there is concomitant compression of the descending aorta at the diaphragm creating a water-hammer effect. This increase in intra-aortic pressure, along with shearing forces on the upper torso where the descending aorta changes from a mobile to a fixed position along the spine, results in the vast majority of aortic injuries being located at the level of the aortic isthmus. Multi-slice CT with multireconstruction will rarely miss an aortic injury. Angiography has a significant role in the management of aortic injury with the endovascular placement of stent graft as the primary choice of repair.

Splenic and hepatic injuries are diagnosed on CT and intervention may be required for evidence of active hepatic bleeding or splenic pseudoaneurysms. Angiography is usually started with a nonselective abdominal aortic angiogram to identify anatomy and potential sites of bleeding followed by selective arteriograms of celiac axis including the liver and spleen, as well as injection of the superior mesenteric artery (SMA) for portal venous studies. Embolization is the treatment of choice if an arterial bleeding source if identified. Multiple views are required before a traumatic arterial injury can be reliable ruled out; in trauma *one view equals no views.*

Severe pelvic injuries are associated with major blood loss which is usually venous in nature. However, 6 % of pelvic bleeding is arterial. If active extravasation is identified on CT, pelvic embolization should be considered prior to operative fixation. The most common pelvic artery injuries include the superior gluteal, iliolumbar, lateral sacral (associated with sacral fracture and sacroiliac joint disruption), internal pudendal, and obturator arteries (associated with pubic rami and acetabular fractures).

10.4.2 Embolization

Embolization is the deliberate blockage of target vessel or territory to stop hemorrhage with minimal nontarget embolization. A thorough knowledge of anatomy and its variants are essential before proceeding. Anatomic anastamoses between vascular territories are particularly important because inflow and outflow will need to be blocked to control bleeding in certain situations and blockage in others will impact adjacent arterial supply with potential disastrous results. The level of embolization also needs to be determined at the onset of the procedure (i.e., treating only the feeding bleeding vessel or the entire vascular bed).

Embolic agents consist of two broad types: temporary or permanent. They are further subdivided into mechanical occlusion (coils, detachable plugs), particulate agents (Gelfoam, polymers), and liquid agents (sclerosants and adhesives). Coils and plugs are permanent agents and are used to occlude specific vessels or pack aneurysms. They work by damage to the intima and provide a large thrombogenic surface and mechanical obstruction of the lumen. Coils are available in a wide array of shapes, diameters, and materials and typically are impregnated with filamentous material to enhance thrombus formation. They may be simply pushed out of the catheter by a guidewire or may be deliverable by specific mechanisms built into the coil allowing certain coils to be removed prior to detachment if placement is determined to be suboptimal. The most important considerations for the operator are whether the coil is compatible with the catheter in place and sized appropriately for the target vessel. Coil thickness is equivalent to guidewire diameter and typically varies from 0.014 to 0.038 in.. Size of the coil (the loops in the coil) and length should be matched to the vessel and task. A coil that is too large in loop diameter will not coil properly and will be straightened in the vessel possibly resulting in catheter displacement. A coil that is too small in loop diameter will migrate distally, potentially to vital nontarget areas (necessitating retrieval). Before delivering the coil, ensure that the catheter is properly position in the target vessel. Standard coils are held straight in a short cartridge which is discarded after the coil is introduced in the catheter. The coil can then be advance into position by a guidewire or dedicated coil pusher. Success is achieved with tight packing of the coils which requires stable catheter position and correctly sized coils. After a few coils are place, perform an angiogram to access flow. If flow is slow, wait a few minutes to see if the vessel thromboses; otherwise continue to carefully pack until flow completely stopped. Once target is coil embolized, distal access through the embolized vessel is no longer possible. Collateral supply to the area of injury must be considered. For this reason, distal access to a pseudoaneurysm, for example, must first be coil embolized ("distal control") before coiling proximally. Post-embolization angiogram should be performed to confirm hemostasis.

Particulate embolic agents are best used when multiple vessels require blockade and target organ tolerance to ischemia is high. These agents are mixed with contrast and injected under direct visualization until flow in the vessel ceases or is markedly diminished. Care must be taken to inject with the right amount of force to avoid reflux. A "6-beat rule" is sometimes used to establish stasis, meaning lack of significant motion of the contrast column for 6 heartbeats is equivalent to appropriate stasis in the vessel. Gelfoam provides temporary occlusion, whereas polymeric particles such as polyvinyl alcohol (PVA) and tris-acryl gel particles (Embospheres®) provide permanent blockage. Gelfoam is available in a powder (40–60 μm) but is most commonly comes in sheets which can be cut into small pledgets and mixed with contrast to form a Gelfoam slurry. Gelfoam is often used in trauma as it can provide nonpermanent hemostasis quickly to a larger vascular bed where a specific bleeding vessel may not be identified. Note that the vascular blockade produced by Gelfoam powder is quite profound and may cause severe injury; the use of Gelfoam powder should be avoided unless the operator is extensively experienced with embolization techniques.

Polymer particle sizes range from 150 to 1,200 μm with particles being provided in bottles with narrower ranges (e.g., 100–300 μm, 300–500 μm). Embospheres™ are compressible spherical particles, approved for use in fibroid embolization. Small particles penetrate the arteriole bed more deeply than larger particles and are more appropriate for tumors. Polymeric particles such as PVA or Embospheres™ are rarely employed in trauma since their small size results in permanent end-arteriole embolization. Reflux from the catheter of these permanent agents can result in disastrous nontarget embolization.

Liquid agents are divided into sclerosants, glues, and thrombin. They are the most difficult to control and least forgiving. Their use should be restricted to the most experienced interventionalists and are beyond the scope of this chapter.

10.5 Clinical Application

10.5.1 Spleen

Embolization for splenic injuries is indicated by the presence of active extravasation and/or pseudoaneurysms. Unlike the liver, the spleen is an end organ and embolization, particularly particulate embolization, could lead to infarct. Proximal versus distal embolization of the spleen remains a somewhat controversial issue. Selective coil embolization is the procedure of choice in controlling small areas of focal intrasplenic bleeding or pseudoaneurysm formation. Due to preserved collaterals from the gastroduodenal, pancreatic, and gastric branches, proximal coiling embolization (of the main splenic artery) is associated with low risk of splenic infarct and is very effective for global, diffuse, or multiple areas of splenic injury. Detachable embolization plugs (e.g., AMPLATZER™ plugs) sized 30–50 % greater than the main vessel diameter or coils can be employed for proximal embolization. Distal coil embolization carries a higher risk of splenic infarct and requires more time to perform. However, selective embolization should be performed for extrasplenic hemorrhage due to the degree of hemodynamic instability and risk of continued bleeding. Both proximal and distal embolization are 90–95 % technically successful; however the observed clinically success rate is closer to 86 % (Figs. 10.3 and 10.4).

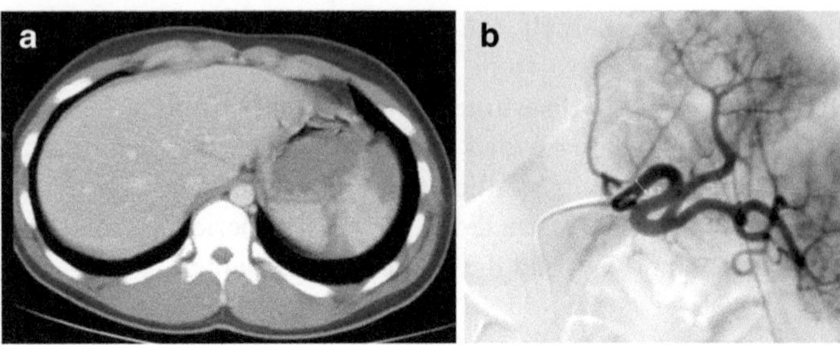

Fig. 10.3 (**a**, **b**) Axial CTA image (**a**) shows grade 4 splenic laceration with surrounding fluid (blood). DSA image (**b**) shows angiogram for sizing of coil size selection. Note there is no active site of bleeding identified. Patient was hemodynamically unstable and therefore proximal embolization was sought

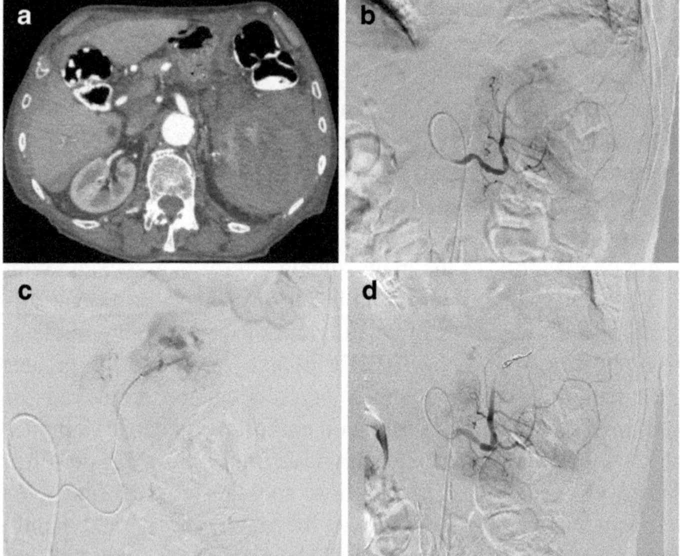

Fig. 10.4 (**a–d**) Axial CTA image shows fluid surrounding the spleen (**a**). DSA image (**b**) with catheter in the splenic artery shows area of active contrast extravasation in the superior portion of the spleen. Selective arteriogram with microcatheter (**c**) confirms branch for target embolization. Post-embolization arteriogram (**d**) shows successful occlusion of the bleeding site

10.5.2   Liver

Blunt hepatic injury is more commonly venous rather than arterial. However, arterial bleeding is usually focal involving small or medium branches and suitable for embolization. Hepatic arteries are not end arteries and there are multiple collaterals. When possible, it is best to start placing coils distal to the injury and working proximal to control bleeding. If unable to get a catheter to the site of injury and the bleed appears is low flow, more proximal embolization with Gelfoam slurry typically will achieve effective hemostasis. Initial embolization with Gelfoam followed by coil embolization is an acceptable alternative. Particle embolization should be distal to the cystic artery when possible as this is the one area within the hepatic circulation that lacks the dual supply typical of the liver. Because of dual supply from the hepatic artery and portal vein, large areas of hepatic embolization are generally well tolerated. However, complications such as high-grade liver injury with abscess formation, hepatic necrosis, or biliary injury (including gallbladder infarction) may occur although these complications can also often be managed by interventional techniques. Focal arterial injuries near the arterial origin can be embolized but covered stents are an attractive alternative when possible (Fig. 10.5).

10.5.3   Kidney

Injuries in the kidney may be to the parenchyma or the vascular pedicle. Arteriovenous fistulas (AVF), pseudoaneurysms, or bleed can occur in either. Embolization in the kidney differs from the spleen and liver as there is no collateral supply in the kidney. Thus, embolization in the kidney will result in infarct and kidney function may be impacted by volume embolized. For this reason, it is desirable to be as selective as possible when

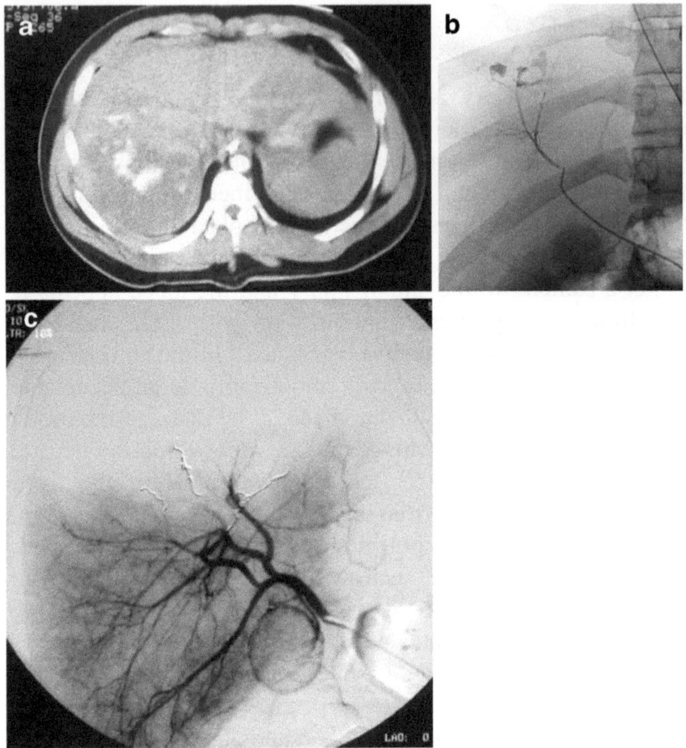

Fig. 10.5 (**a–c**) Axial CTA image (**a**) showing active bleed in the liver. DSA image (**b**) through the 5 Fr catheter shows multiple areas of active extravasation from multiple vessels. Selective embolization through a microcatheter was performed. (**c**) Post-embolization DSA image shows occlusion of multiple bleeding vessels with coils

attempting to embolize renal arteries. Main artery injury can be treated with a covered stent in some cases. Selective coil embolization is preferred for intraparenchymal injury when a focal bleeding artery can be identified. Gelfoam or particles can be used for more distal injury (Fig. 10.6).

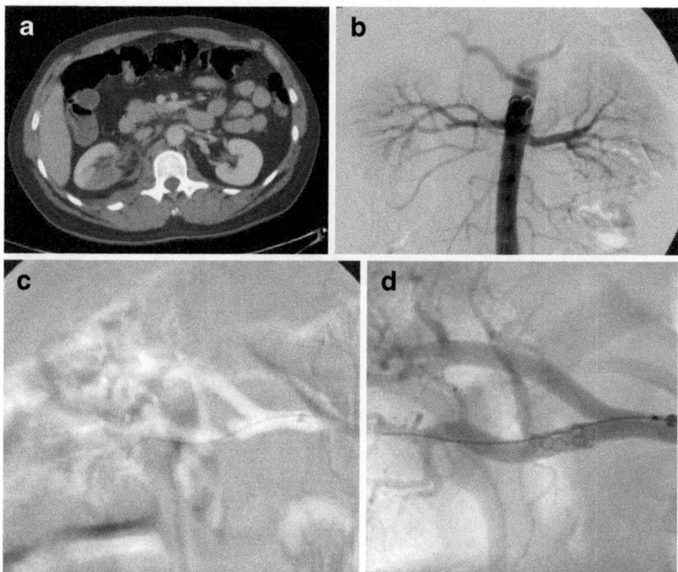

Fig. 10.6 (**a–d**) Axial CTA (**a**) shows perfusion defect in the right kidney. DSA image (**b**) demonstrates a notched appearance in the inferior renal artery. Image from the "road map" function (**c**) where the operator sees an overlay of the vessel was used to position a stent across the dissection. (**d**) Post-stenting angiogram shows successful restoration of flow in the artery

10.5.4 Pelvis

Bleeding from major pelvic trauma is typically venous and often will subside with placement of a pelvic binder. However, arterial bleeding will not usually respond to this intervention. The arterial bleeding almost invariably lies over the fracture site. Even minor fractures particularly in the elderly can be associated with major arterial hemorrhage and should be taken into consideration in their traumatic evaluation. Overall, pelvic embolization is successful in treating hemorrhage in 85–90 % of cases.

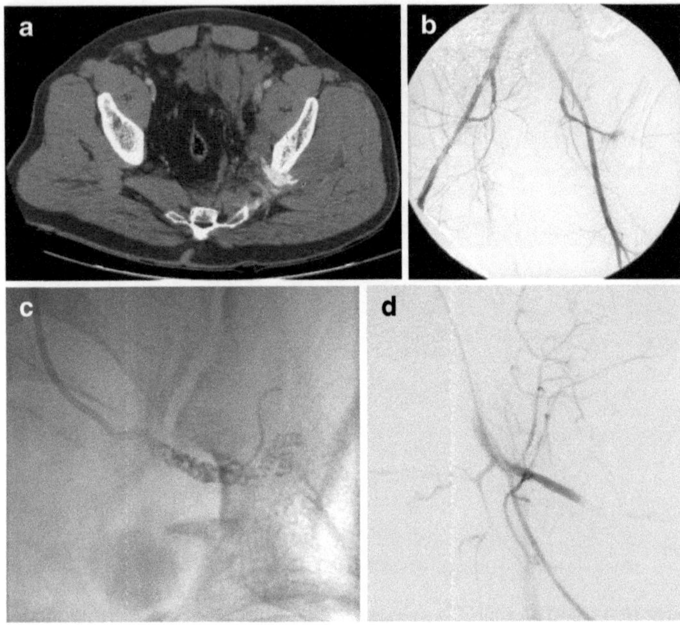

Fig. 10.7 (**a–d**) Axial CTA image (**a**) shows contrast extravasation in the left hemipelvis between the sacrum and the ilium. DSA (**b**) shows corresponding bleed from the internal iliac artery. Coil embolization ensued (**c**) with successful hemostasis (**d**)

Selective arteriograms of the internal iliac artery should be performed for pelvic trauma. Superselective embolization with coils (preferred), Gelfoam, or rarely particles can be performed. If there are multiple areas of extravasation, nonselective embolization of the anterior or posterior division or even the internal iliac artery itself can be performed with Gelfoam as an extreme measure. Risks of pelvic embolization are increased however with this maneuver including uterine/prostate/bladder necrosis, paresis, impotence, and buttock ischemia (Fig. 10.7).

10.5.5   Extremity

Extremity arterial trauma most often accompanies orthopedic injuries. Fractures and dislocations may result in injury, including after reduction. Revascularization with surgical bypass is the mainstay, but occasionally a stent graft can bridge a dissection. More typically an occlusion balloon can stop hemorrhage until surgical repair. Embolization can be carried out safely in the muscular branches of the arm or leg due to collateral supply. This collateral supply is more effective proximal to the knee and elbow compared to the distal extremities. Provided the palmar arch is intact, injuries to one of the interosseous, radial, or ulnar arteries can be performed with coils. Particles are contraindicated due to distal embolization risk in the hand. For the lower extremities, the popliteal artery is most often injured and repair is surgical. The common femoral and superficial femoral arteries cannot be embolized (nor can their supply, the common/external iliac arteries). The profunda femoris branches can be safely embolized due to collateral supply. Because of this collateral supply, proximal and distal control at the site of injury should be sought. Isolated injuries to one of the runoff vessels can be coil embolized provided the plantar arch is patent. Because of this collateral pathway, again proximal and distal control is warranted (Fig. 10.8).

10.5.6   Large Vessel (Aorta)

Aortic dissections and transections can be successfully managed with endovascular techniques. Endovascular management of with covered stents/grafts is covered elsewhere in this text.

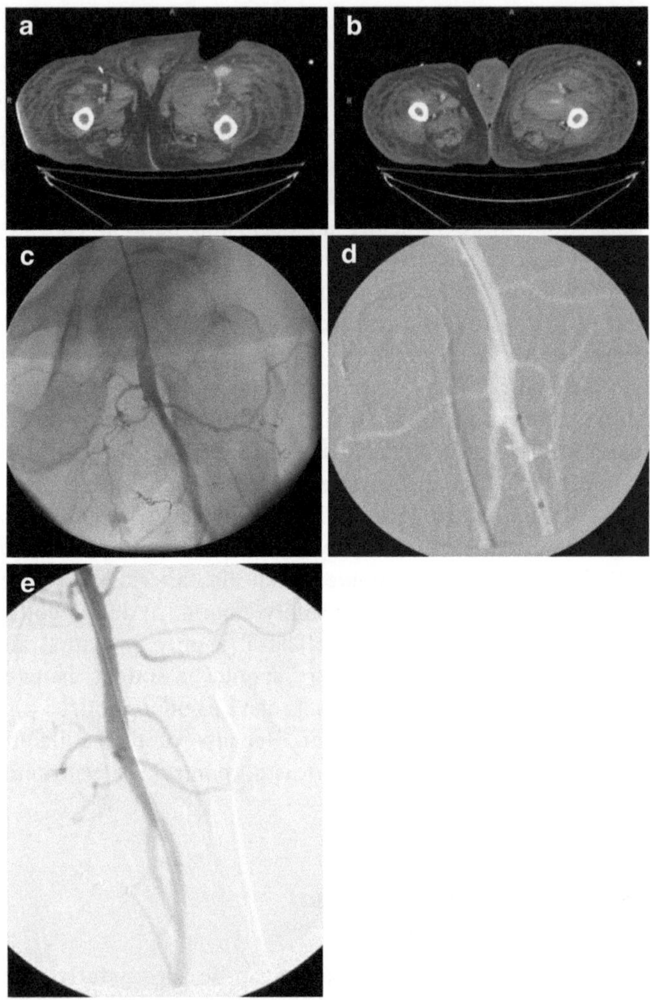

Fig. 10.8 Axial CTA images show bleeds in the region of the superficial femoral artery (**a**) and profunda femoral artery (**b**). DSA image (**c**) after coiling the profunda branch bleed shows persistent extravasation which was identified to be arising from an SFA. Because this was not amenable to coiling, a covered stent was positioned (**d**) to exclude the bleed. Post-embolization DSA (**e**) shows resolution of the bleed

10.5.7   Advancing Technology

Endovascular techniques have gained wide acceptance in the management of peripheral vascular disease, aortic aneurysms, and aortic dissections. However, there is increasing evidence that these same techniques have a role in the management of trauma vascular injury and hemorrhagic shock. Endovascular balloon occlusion, temporary hemorrhage control, and stenting of traumatic injured great and proximal peripheral vessels have been published in case reports and small series. Additionally, aortic balloon occlusion has been shown to have a clear benefit in the management of rupture abdominal aortic aneurysm.

Resuscitative endovascular balloon occlusion of the aorta (REBOA) is being evaluated as an alternate to the resuscitative thoracotomy for traumatic arrest or impending trauma arrest from hemorrhagic shock. Endovascular balloon occlusion has a significant advantage over resuscitative thoracotomy by limiting the secondary insult to a patient already in extremis. The technique could be applied in the trauma bay with or without fluoroscopy. Access is obtained via the femoral artery with a puncture needle, and a 0.035 in guidewire is advanced into the femoral and iliac artery. An initial 5–8 Fr sheath is passed over the wire. Balloon used for aortic occlusion must be compliant and large enough to occlude significant antegrade flow. Examples of balloons would be the Coda® 14 Fr (Cook Medical), Reliant® 12 Fr (Medtronic, Inc.), and Berenstein™ 6 Fr (Boston Scientific). The balloon sheaths need to be placed over a much stiffer and longer wire (180 cm). The placement of this stiffer wire requires fluoroscopy due to the increased risk of vascular injury. Once the stiffer wire is placed, the initial sheath can be removed and a larger sheath which can accommodate the balloon is advanced over the wire into the aortic position. The balloon is loaded on the wire and advanced to the end of the larger sheath. Inflation of the balloon should be accomplished under fluoroscopy. A 30–60 cc syringe filled with 50/50 saline/contrast is used to inflate the balloon. The balloon is inflated until the outer edges change from convex to parallel. Once inflated, the balloon, sheath, and wire must be secured to the patient. Once the device is no longer required, the balloon and wire can be removed. The large sheath is best removed by surgical exploration with closure of the arteriotomy.

10.6 Summary

- Diagnostic angiography for trauma is rare in the setting of modern CTA. Most angiography is undertaken with the intent for intervention; however, diagnostic angiography still begins all procedures.
- Multiple agents exist for transcatheter embolization of arterial hemorrhage. Choice of the appropriate embolic agent (e.g., coils, gelfoam, particles) depends on the clinical scenario and the expertise and experience of the interventionalist.
- Because arterial bleeding can lead to coagulopathy, embolization is best performed early as agents such as coils and particles are designed to be thombogenic.
- Stent grafts are a mainstay for aortic injury and smaller grafts can sometimes be used to for smaller vessels.
- Multidisciplinary teams with established protocols for trauma are fundamental for deciding which patients are appropriate for embolization versus surgical intervention.

Suggesting Reading

Glorsky SL, Wonderlich DA, Goei AD (2010) Evaluation and management of the trauma patient for the interventional radiologist. Semin Interv Radiol 27(1):29–37

Gruen RL, Brohi K, Schreiber M, Balogh ZJ, Pitt V, Narayan M, Maier RV (2012) Haemorrhage control in severely injured patients. Lancet 380(9847):1099–1108

Howell GM, Peitzman AB, Nirula R, Rosengart MR, Alarcon LH, Billiar TR, Sperry JL (2010) Delay to therapeutic interventional radiology postinjury: time is of the essence. J Trauma 68(6):1296–1300

Kessel D, Robertson I (2011) Interventional radiology a survival guide, 3rd edn. Elsevier, Edinburgh

Salazar GM, Walker TG (2009) Evaluation and management of acute vascular trauma. Tech Vasc Interv Radiol 12(2):102–116

Stannard A, Eliason JL, Rasmussen TE (2011) Resuscitative endovascular balloon occlusion of the aorta (REBOA) as an adjunct for hemorrhagic shock. J Trauma 71(6):1869–1872

Zealley IA, Chakraverty S (2010) The role of interventional radiology in trauma. BMJ 8:350

Chapter 11
Management of Penetrating Neck Injuries

Patrizio Petrone, Juan M. Verde, and Juan A. Asensio

P. Petrone, MD (⊠)
Department of Surgery, Hospital General 'Prof. Dr. Luis Güemes',
University of Buenos Aires School of Medicine,
San Martín 2544 – 4° "A", Mar del Plata (7600) – Prov. of Bs. As.,
Argentina

Ministry of Health, La Plata, Prov. of Buenos Aires, Argentina
e-mail: patrizio.petrone@gmail.com

J.M. Verde, MD
Gastrointestinal Surgery Division, Hospital de Clínicas,
University of Buenos Aires School of Medicine,
Córdoba 2351, 7° floor, Ciudad Autónoma de
Buenos Aires CABA 1425, Argentina
e-mail: juanmaverde@juanmaverde.com.ar

J.A. Asensio, MD, FACS, FCCM
Department of Surgery, New York Medical College,
Taylor Pavilion, 100 Woods Road, Suite E-137,
Valhalla, NY 10595, USA

Trauma Surgery, Westchester University Medical Center,
Westchester, NY, USA
e-mail: asensioj@wcmc.com

S. Di Saverio et al. (eds.), *Trauma Surgery*,
DOI 10.1007/978-88-470-5403-5_11, © Springer-Verlag Italia 2014

11.1   Introduction

Penetrating injuries of the neck were always considered difficult to manage, mostly because of a dense concentration of vital structures contained in a very small body area. Many of these structures are difficult to examine and technically challenging to expose.

The controversy between initial surgical management and a selective conservative approach still exists. This chapter discusses the initial evaluation of penetrating neck injuries and its historical evolution, aiming to offer guidelines in the management of specific complex injuries.

11.2   Historical Perspective

The first documented case of the treatment of a cervical vascular injury is attributed to the French military surgeon Ambroise Paré, who ligated the lacerated carotid artery and jugular vein of a wounded French soldier [1]. In 1803, Fleming [2] ligated the lacerated common carotid artery of a sailor, with a successful outcome, and in 1811, Abernathy [3] ligated the lacerated left common and internal carotid arteries in a patient who sustained an injury by a bull.

The military setting during wartime has always provided the surgeon with an opportunity to advance the science of trauma surgery. In armed conflicts, mortality rates ranged from 7 % during World War II to 15 % in the Vietnam conflict, while in the civilian arena is reported to range from 0 to 11 % [4–8].

In 1944, Bailey [9] proposed early exploration of all cervical hematomas, and in 1956, Fry and Fry [10] showed a 6 % mortality rate in patients undergoing early neck explorations versus a 35 % mortality rate in those patients not immediately managed surgically or undergoing exploration on a delayed basis. They also demonstrated an increase in the mortality rate in those patients explored after 6 h, and based on that, they advocated early exploration of every neck injury violating the platysma.

As time elapsed, the rates of negative neck explorations range from 40 to 63 %. Thus the concept of selective management seeks to identify through various diagnostic criteria those patients who would benefit from early surgical intervention.

The contrast became evident. On the one hand, the consequences of missed injury with the very low morbidity of neck exploration and, on the other hand, the selective exploration demonstrate a decrease in the rate of negative neck exploration with equally good outcomes [11].

11.3 Anatomy

The neck represents the narrowest section of the axial body, designed to protect and allow for the vital structures to connect the head to the trunk. The cervical region is limited above by the mandible, mastoid processes, and superior nuchal line and below by the sternum, clavicles, and cervical seventh' spinous processes.

Deep into the skin lies the subcutaneous tissue and superficial layer of the cervical fascia that splits to surround the sternocleidomastoid and trapezius muscles. The pretracheal layer contains some hyoid muscles, and the prevertebral fascia includes the homonymous muscles.

The midsection of the neck hosts the aerodigestive components, and it descends into the thorax along with the neck nerves and vessels that run along each side. This section includes the carotid arteries (CA) and internal jugular vein (IJV). These structures lie superficially immediately under the skin, protected only by the vertebrae posteriorly. This makes them vulnerable to any penetrating injuries, as opposed to the skull and chest that encase their vital organs. It is very important to remember that the vertebral arteries go through the transverse foramen along the cervical column on their way into the skull and they are positioned lateral to the major anterior vessels.

The classic categorization of the neck's anatomical sections in terms of the variable consequences of penetrating trauma divides the region in three anatomical zones with both sternocleidomastoid muscles as lateral limits [12]. Zone I ranges from the level of the clavicles and sternal notch inferiorly to the cricoid cartilage above. The proximal CA, IJV, and subclavian vessels are the most important vascular structures of this zone, which also include lungs (apical segments), esophagus, trachea, and thoracic duct. Zone II extends from the cricoid cartilage to the angle of the mandible; included here are the longer portions of the neck vessels (CA and IJVs), as well as the larynx and hypopharynx. Injuries in the zone III are limited to the area between the angle of mandible and base of the skull. The superior segment of cervical vessels can be damaged fast turning into a challenge for the surgeon in charge.

Zone II is the largest and therefore the most affected one. On the other hand it is more accessible and easier to evaluate, thus suitable for simple and fast surgical exposure. This is not the case for zones I and III, as they require the use of complementary studies in order to decide upon the best approach and correct treatment. They are both difficult to approach and result much more challenging for the surgeon.

Thorough evaluation and knowledge of the neck anatomy is crucial for the trauma surgeon, who needs to assess promptly the correct initial evaluation and management of the patient, having considered the location of the lesion and the proximity of those vital elements surrounding it.

11.4 Evaluation and Diagnosis

Clinical manifestations depend on the neck structure(s) involved in the injury; they can be very heterogeneous, ranging from totally asymptomatic to polysymptomatic patients. Hence, a neck evaluation should be performed in any trauma victim in order to discard vascular or cervical spinal lesions.

Initial evaluation must attend to the presence of "hard signs" of neck injury that are mostly related with vessel injuries and demand urgent surgical intervention. These are, for example, the presence of an expanding and/or pulsatile hematoma or brisk bleeding from the wound, bruit, or thrill. The hard signs are usually associated to pulse deficit and cerebral ischemia with neurological signs or symptoms [13].

Recognition of other findings in the absence of "hard signs" is included in the group of "soft signs." The most common ones are hemoptysis/hematemesis, oropharyngeal blood, nonexpanding hematoma, dysphonia/dysphagia, subcutaneous or mediastinal emphysema, and focal neurologic deficits. A more selective approach is mandatory for these patients (arteriography or Doppler ultrasonography, esophagoscopy, laryngoscopy, or tracheoscopy).

Potential injuries must be evaluated by careful assessment of pulses, bruits, size and expansion of hematomas, and any neurological findings suggesting vascular injury related to ischemia. Penetrating injuries can never be assessed by examination of the local extension of the wound in the emergency room. Exploration should be performed in the operating room by a formal neck surgical exploration.

The proper diagnosis of the unstable patients sustaining penetrating injuries should be performed intraoperatively by means of a formal exploration. Hemorrhagic shock, stroke, unstable airway, and expanding hematoma are also indications of surgical exploration. In stable patients with penetrating neck injuries, the physical examination and x-rays are the usual initial tests.

Emphysema is often the most common indicator of an aerodigestive injury and is evident on neck x-ray studies. The lowest structures as the larynx may present with cervicofacial emphysema when disrupted, whereas when the trachea is the one affected, massive mediastinal and deep cervical emphysema may be observed.

The multidetector computed tomography (MDCT) is a method that accurately identifies the extrapulmonary air and locates the affected structure. In rare cases indirect signs of tracheal wall disruptions can be noted and diagnosed (i.e., tracheal tube balloon herniation).

In the second stage of a selective approach, we can use the flexible laryngoscopy, esophagoscopy, and bronchoscopy that are intended to diagnose aerodigestive injuries. An early diagnosis of esophageal injury is usually very difficult. Despite a negative CT, if there is a high suspicion of esophageal injury, flexible esophagoscopy with or without esophagography should be performed to rule it out and prevent fulminant mediastinitis, which is associated to high mortality.

In asymptomatic and stable patients with penetrating injuries located in zones I and III, the arteriography remains the gold standard for the evaluation of the cervical vessels. Similar sensitivity and specificity is achieved by angio-CT with MDCT and a correct intravenous bolus of contrast. Although stable, any patient with zone II neck injury that presents with persistent hemorrhage or neurological deficits compatible with adjacent vascular damage (i.e., Horner's syndrome) should be evaluated by angiography.

It is important to know that patients with negative arteriography results and positive physical examination still need surgical exploration. Color flow Doppler ultrasonography is noninvasive and convenient, but the sensitivity for vascular injury is highly operator dependent. When performed by experienced technicians, the sensitivity has been reported to be 90–95 % for injuries requiring surgical intervention [14].

11.5 Management Principles

The advanced trauma life support (ATLS®) should be the initial guideline for the management of penetrating neck injuries. These guidelines establish priorities in diagnostics and treatment of life-threatening injuries.

Up to 10 % of penetrating neck injuries involve the airway [15]. This compromise may be due to direct trauma, large hematoma compressing the airway, or airway edema. A pathognomonic sign of airway injury is air bubbling through a neck injury. Manual compression increases oxygenation by reducing the air leak. It is important that the management of the airway must be done by a trained physician since the key point of this situation is to rapidly determine the need of endotracheal intubation or an emergent surgical airway.

Endotracheal intubation should be the initial approach of airway injuries, and this procedure must be done by an operator trained in advanced management of airway. Emergent surgical airway is reserved for cases in which the endotracheal intubation seems to be difficult due to anatomic or injury considerations. The use of fiber-optic intubation could be helpful, but it requires training and it has a failure rate of 20 % as described in the literature [15]. Cricothyroidotomy is the gold standard procedure for surgical management of the airway. It can be easily and rapidly performed, but its difficulty increases during the presence of large neck hematomas.

Control of hemorrhage is the second major topic that has to be mention. In most cases external bleeding can easily be controlled by direct pressure. However, in certain anatomical locations like below the base of the skull, the vertebral artery topography, and behind the clavicle, this control by direct pressure is difficult to achieve. In this situation, the use of a finger or a balloon catheter to control hemorrhage may be helpful. Blind clamping is rarely effective and should be avoided because of the potential damage to other structures.

11.6 Specific Injuries

11.6.1 Carotid Artery Injuries

Carotid artery injuries are the most difficult and certainly the most immediate life-threatening injuries found in penetrating neck trauma. Their potential for causing fatal neurological outcomes, their propensity to bleed actively, and

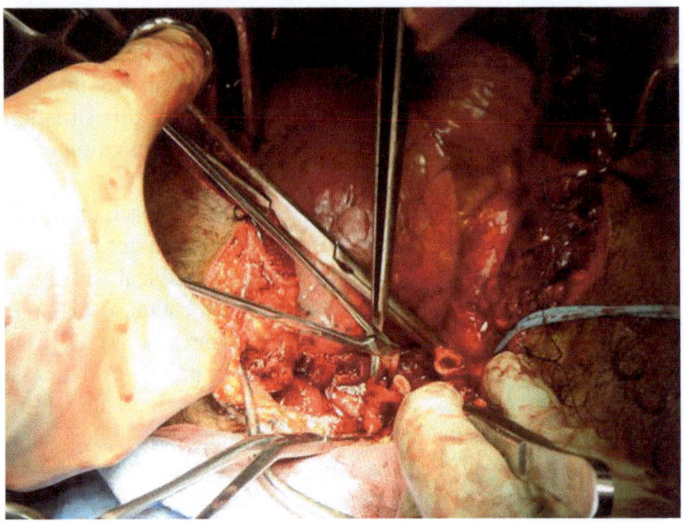

Fig. 11.1 Left intrathoracic carotid artery secondary to gunshot wound

their potential to occlude the airway demand a rapid response by the trauma team.

Carotid artery injuries are estimated to be present in 6–13 % of all penetrating injuries to the neck [11]. Asensio has reported an incidence of 11–13 % carotid artery injuries for all penetrating neck injuries [11]. Penetrating is the most frequent mechanism of injury (Fig. 11.1).

The majority of carotid artery injuries are confined to the common carotid artery. According to the literature, the carotid artery segment that most frequently is involved is the common carotid (73 %), followed by the internal carotid (22 %), and finally the external carotid (5 %) [16].

For the operative management of carotid artery injury, the patient should be placed in supine position on the operating table with the head facing the contralateral side of the injury. The face, neck, supraclavicular area, and thoracic area must be

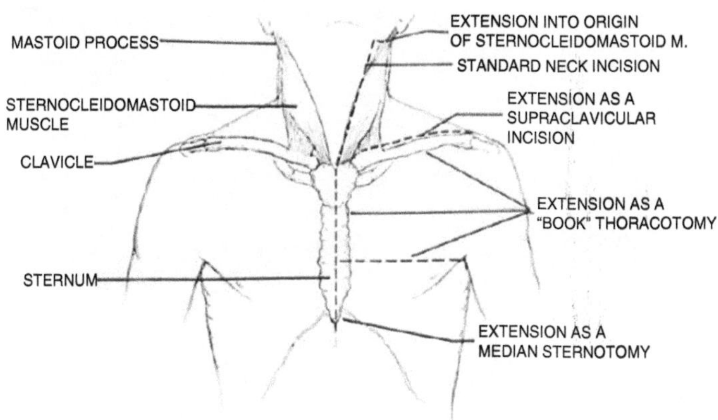

Fig. 11.2 Incisions [11]

included in the operating field. The contralateral groin should be also prepared in case a saphenous vein graft is needed to repair the carotid injury. The neck should be explored by a standard incision in the anterior border of the sternocleidomastoid (SCM) muscle, from the angle of the mandible up to the sternoclavicular junction (Fig. 11.2). Below the SCM muscle the internal jugular vein can be found. Medially deeper to it, the carotid artery can be found. The facial vein is usually transected in order to expose the common carotid bifurcation. Once exposed it is essential to obtain proximal and distal control of the common, internal, and external sections of the carotid artery.

If the injury is possible for primary repair, lateral arteriorrhaphy should be attempted. However, in injuries that produced extensive destruction of the carotid artery, resection of the involved segment should be done followed by reconstruction of the artery. End-to-end primary anastomosis can be done (Fig. 11.3) if there is no sign of tension. If this occurs, the interposition of a saphenous vein graft should be performed (Fig. 11.4). As an option, instead of a saphenous vein graft, a PTFE graft can be

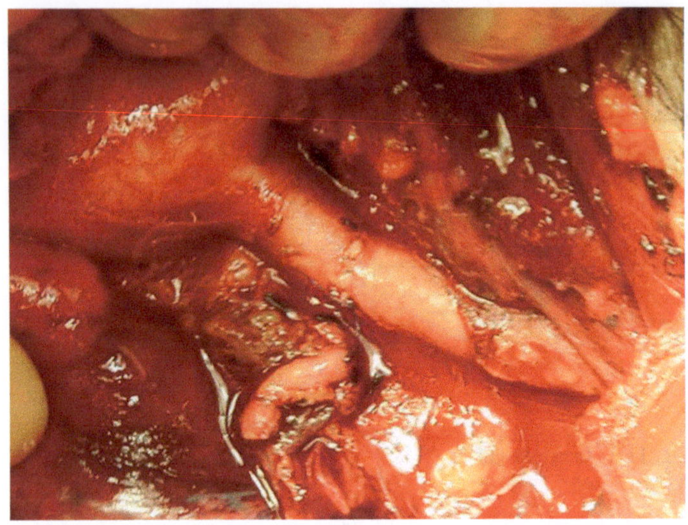

Fig. 11.3 Primary repair performing end-to-end anastomosis

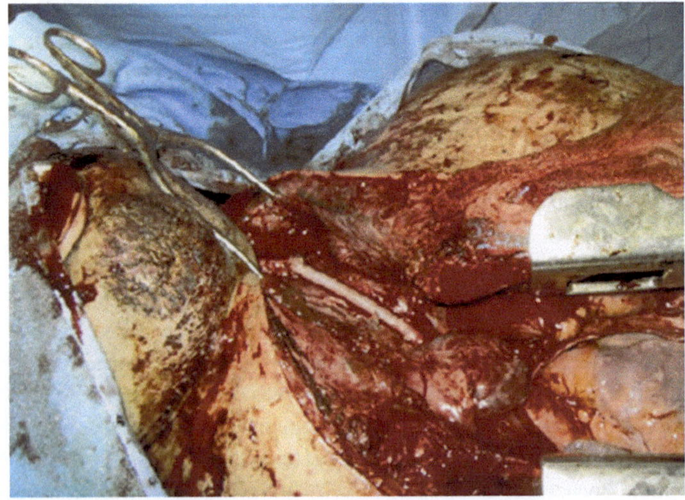

Fig. 11.4 Carotid repair with autogenous saphenous vein

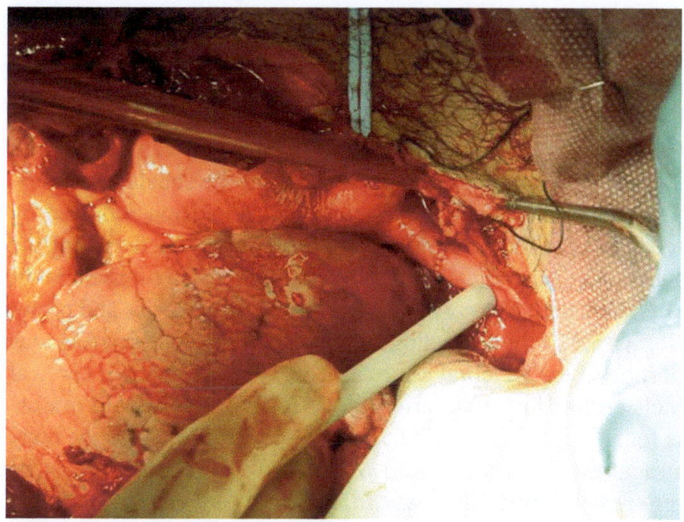

Fig. 11.5 Pulse checked by a handheld Doppler probe

used in order to restore blood flow. Doppler signal analysis should be performed after the repair is complete (Fig. 11.5). The use of 5,000 units of heparin systematically is recommended in this type of injuries [16].

11.6.2   *Vertebral Artery Injuries*

Vertebral artery injuries are uncommon and usually they are not life-threatening. The incidence of these injuries varies from 1 % up to 7.4 % [17]. The most common mechanisms of injuries are gunshot wounds, followed by stab wounds. These injuries are often associated to other injuries such as aerodigestive injuries, cervical spine, nerve injuries, and other vascular injuries. According to Rowe et al., associated vascular injuries occur in a range from 13 to 19 % [17].

The vast majority of vertebral artery injuries does not require any treatment or are treated with angiography. The operative management of these injuries is reserved for patients with active bleeding or those that angiographic treatment had failed. Proximal vascular control of the vertebral artery can be achieved at the base of the neck where it comes off the subclavian artery. This approach requires a supraclavicular incision followed by transection of the SCM muscle off the clavicle. By retracting the subclavian vein caudally and the anterior scalene muscle laterally, the vertebral artery can be found in the superior and posterior aspect of the ascending subclavian artery. The interosseous portion of the vertebral artery is achieved by a standard cervical incision like in carotid artery injuries. The longus colli muscle is found deep in the neck and should be removed from the bony structures. The anterior rim of the vertebral foramen must be removed in order to expose the vertebral artery. The vertebral artery can be safely ligated without major complications. Special care must be taken in order to avoid injury to the nerves. It is important to remark that the preferred approach of these injuries is angiographically.

11.6.3 *Laryngotracheal Injuries*

Laryngotracheal injuries are uncommon injuries. They are present in 1/30,000 emergency room visits. In penetrating neck injuries the incidence of laryngotracheal injury varies between 2 and 4 % [17]. The management of these injuries varies from nonoperative management up to operative management, but most of these injuries are beneficiated with early operative intervention. Besides hemodynamic support, oxygenation and ventilation of these patients are important.

Airway injuries are challenging even for experienced surgeons. These injuries can be approach by a transverse incision that can be extended caudal or cephalad along the midline according to the extension of the injury. When the injury involves the distal trachea or the carina, median sternotomy is needed. Small laryngotracheal injuries can be primarily repair with absorbable sutures. More extensive injuries require debridement and end-to-end anastomosis. The key point is to perform a tension-free anastomosis. Mobilization of the airway must be done in the anterior and posterior aspects since vascular supply runs sideways of the trachea. When both tracheal ends are less than three centimeters away, primary anastomosis can be achieved. If the defect is greater, mobilization of the larynx and flexion of the neck are required. After the repair, the neck should be maintained in flexion for at least 1 week by suturing the chin to the chest. In patients with instability, tracheostomy alone is utilized, postponing the definite repair of the airway.

11.6.4 Pharyngoesophageal Injuries

Digestive tract injuries are rare. Since these injuries are not immediate life-threatening, associated injuries are high priority. Signs and symptoms of pharyngoesophageal injuries, such as odynophagia, subcutaneous emphysema, or hematemesis, are found in less than 25 % of patients, and less than 20 % of patients presenting these symptoms have a digestive tract injury [18].

Prompt repair of these injuries during the first 24 h decreases the incidence of septic complications. The exposure of the pharynx and esophagus is achieved by a standard cervicotomy. The vascular component of the neck are retracted laterally and the airway medially. Injuries by gunshot wound require debridement. The repair can be performed in one layer of absorbable suture or two layers with absorbable sutures in the first layer and nonabsorbable sutures in the second layer. External diversion is reserved for injuries associated with abscess and infection.

11.7 Conclusions

The greatest advances in injury management are always made during wars. During the Civil War, observation was the mainstay of treatment, which carried 15 % mortality. During World War I, observation still a valid approach at that time, with sporadic exploration and ligation, and the mortality ranged from 11 to 18 %. But during World War II, things started to change to mandatory exploration and attempts to vascular repairs, with a subsequent drop in mortality rates to 7 %. During the Korean and Vietnam conflicts, mandatory exploration and vascular repair were common practice, but the mortality increased to 15 %, mainly due to the use of a more sophisticated weapons. In the civilian arena, mandatory exploration has been replaced by selective management, with mortality rates ranging from 0 to 11 % [19].

We can conclude that a selective approach is safe in the asymptomatic and hemodynamically stable patient, provided that accurate diagnostic means are immediately available to exclude injuries needing immediate surgical management. Also, the mandatory approach is a safe, reliable, and time-tested method of dealing with these injuries.

On the basis of the current review of the literature, we cannot recommend one approach as superior to the other. Once diagnosed, the patient's clinical condition guides treatment. The surgeon has to tailor the approach on the basis of personal as well as institutional experience and the demographics of the patient population served.

References

1. Key G (ed) (1957) The Apologie and Treatise of Ambroise Paré containing the voyages made into divers places with many writings upon surgery. Falcon Education Books, London

2. Fleming D (1817) Case of rupture of the carotid artery and wounds of several of its branches, successfully treated by tying the common trunk of the carotid itself. Med Chir J Rev 3:2

3. Unger SW, Tucker WS Jr, Mrdeza MA, Wellons HA Jr, Chandler JG (1980) Carotid arterial trauma. Surgery 87(5):477–487

4. Beebe GW, DeBakey ME (1952) Battle casualties: incidence, mortality and logistic considerations. Charles C Thomas, Springfield

5. La Garde LA (1916) Gunshot injuries. W. Wood, New York, p 204

6. Ford JH (1927) Medical Department of the United States Army in the World War, vol 2 US Government Printing Office, Washington, DC, p 68

7. Meyer JP, Barrett JA, Schuler JJ, Flanigan DP (1987) Mandatory vs selective exploration for penetrating neck trauma. A prospective assessment. Arch Surg 122(5):592–597

8. Otis GA (1883) Medical and surgical history of the War of Rebellion. In: Surgical history, part 3, vol 2. US Government Printing Office, Washington, DC, p 69

9. Bailey H (1944) Surgery of modern warfare, vol 2, 3rd edn. Williams & Wilkins, Baltimore, p 674

10. Fry RE, Fry WJ (1980) Extracranial carotid artery injuries. Surgery 88(4):581–587

11. Asensio JA, Valenziano CP, Falcone RE, Grosh JD (1991) Management of penetrating neck injuries. Surg Clin North Am 71(2):267–296

12. Demetriades D, Asensio JA, Velmahos G, Thal E (1996) Complex penetrating neck injuries. In: Asensio JA, Demetriades D, Berne TV (eds). W.B. Saunders Co., Philadelphia. Surg Clin North Am 76(4): 685–724

13. Demetriades D, Theodorou D, Cornwell E, Beme TV, Asensio JA, Belzberg H, Velmahos G, Weaver F, Yellin A (1997) Evaluation of penetrating injuries of the neck: prospective study of 223 patients. World J Surg 21(1):41–48

14. Kuma SR, Weaver FA, Yellin AE (2002) Cervical vascular injuries. Carotid and jugular venous injuries. In: Asensio JA, Demetriades D, Feliciano DV, Hoyt DV (eds) W.B. Saunders Co., Philadelphia. Surg Clin North Am 81(6):1331–1344

15. Weireter LJ, Britt LD (2008) Penetrating neck injuries: diagnosis and selective management. In: Asensio JA, Trunkey D (eds) Current therapy of trauma and surgical critical care, 5th edn. Mosby/Elsevier, Philadelphia, pp 197–202

16. Asensio JA, Vu T, Mazzini F, Herrerias F, Pust GD, Sciarretta J, Chandler J, Verde JM, Menendez P, Sanchez JM, Petrone P, Marini C (2011) Penetrating carotid artery: uncommon complex and lethal injuries. Eur J Trauma Emerg Surg 37(5):429–437

17. Rowe V, Petrone P, García-Nuñez LM, Asensio JA (2008) Carotid, vertebral artery, and jugular venous injuries. In: Asensio JA, Trunkey D (eds) Current therapy of trauma and surgical critical care, 5th edn. Mosby/Elsevier, Philadelphia, pp 203–206
18. Demetriades D, Velmahos GG, Asensio JA (2001) Cervical pharyngo-esophageal and laryngotracheal injuries. World J Surg 25(8):1044–1048
19. Asensio JA, Verde JM, Ünlü A, Pust D, Nabri M, Karsidag T, Petrone P (2011) Vascular injuries of the neck. In: Oestern HJ, Trentz O, Uranues S (eds) European Manual of Medicine. Head, thoracic, abdominal, and vascular injuries, 1st edn. Springer, Berlin, pp 381–392

Chapter 12
Acute Traumatic Brain Injuries and Their Management

Michael M. Krausz, Itamar Ashkenazi, and Jean F. Soustiel

Traumatic brain injuries (TBIs) represent the leading cause of death and morbidity in western countries. Since motor vehicle accidents are the leading cause of significant trauma, TBIs affect mostly young adults with increasing incidence and are

M.M. Krausz, MD (⊠)
Shock and Trauma Research Laboratory,
Faculty of Medicine, Technion – Israel Institute
of Technology, Haifa, Israel

Department of Surgery B, Hillel Yaffe Medical Center,
POB 169, Hadera 38100, Israel
e-mail: michaelkrausz100@gmail.com

I. Ashkenazi, MD
Acute Brain Injury Research Laboratory,
Faculty of Medicine, Technion – Israel Institute
of Technology, Haifa, Israel

Department of Surgery B, Hillel Yaffe Medical Center,
POB 169, Hadera 38100, Israel
e-mail: itamara@hy.health.gov.il

J.F. Soustiel, MD
Department of Neurosurgery,
Western Galilee Medical Center, Naharia, Israel
e-mail: j_soustiel@rambam.health.gov.il

S. Di Saverio et al. (eds.), *Trauma Surgery*,
DOI 10.1007/978-88-470-5403-5_12, © Springer-Verlag Italia 2014

responsible for a major social and economic burden. For decades, the mainstay of neurotrauma management has been represented by control of posttraumatic edema and raised intracranial pressure (ICP). With the emergence of a better understanding of the underlying cellular mechanisms responsible for the generation of secondary brain damage, the hope for the "magic bullet" has prompted the development of novel drugs. Encouraged by the promising results of basic research studies, clinical trials were initiated in an increasing number up to the mid-1990s. However, the high expectations raised by convincing laboratory data were not met by deceiving results that made pharmaceutical industry reluctant to support high-cost adventurous research that have repeatedly failed to significantly improve outcome of head-injured patients [1]. Accordingly, the management of neurotrauma has focused back on optimization of neurointensive care and surgical treatment.

12.1 Epidemiology

Although the exact incidence of TBI is difficult to determine as it depends on several criteria such as definition of TBI and the need for hospitalization, a rough estimate is that 1.7 million sustain some form of TBI every year in the USA; of these approximately 1.4 million were treated and released from emergency departments, and 275,000 were hospitalized and discharged alive [2]. Although 75 % of TBIs are concussion or another form of mild brain injury, they are nevertheless responsible for more than 50,000 yearly deaths and one-third of all injury-related death in the USA. TBIs are three times more common in men than in women and occur with the highest incidence in young adults mostly as the result of motor vehicle accidents in western countries and in the elderly as the result of fall [2].

12.2 Biomechanics and Mechanisms of Brain Injuries

Two different types of biomechanical forces can be distinguished: static and dynamic load. These forces, either applied separately or, more commonly, in association, are responsible for contact and inertial types of brain injuries: focal, diffuse, blast, and penetrating.

Contact injuries are created by forces applied to the skull without any associated movement of the head. Since most instances of contact loading to the head will eventually result in some motion, pure form of contact injuries is rare and is characterized by slowly applied forces resulting in focal injuries, either at the impact site or remote from it. According to the energy delivered at the point of impact, the site of the injury in respect to the skull, the size and shape of the stroking object, the direction and magnitude of the stroking force, the extent of the traumatic lesions in terms of severity, and involved structures will vary considerably.

Inertial injuries on the opposite represent the consequence of a dynamic load to the head, either applied without any direct impact to the head (impulsive load) or, more commonly, as a consequence of a fast blow to the head (impact load). In both instances, the head is set in motion, generating acceleration and deceleration forces responsible for strain applied to the brain parenchyma and related vessels, causing functional or structural damage according to the intensity and direction of the applied forces. In this situation, brain damage represents the consequence of differential movements of the brain within the skull on one hand and between different brain structures on the other. Differential movements of the brain within the skull are due to the presence of a physiological subarachnoid compartment around the brain allowing some movement causing surface lesions to neural tissue and cerebral vessels at points of particular susceptibility such as the frontal and temporal regions, either at the point of impact (coup) or on the opposite side (contrecoup). Strain within the brain parenchyma, on the other hand, generates shearing forces responsible for widespread tissue damage involving mostly axons particularly vulnerable to strain and tensile forces [3].

12.3 Pathophysiology of Traumatic Brain Injury

12.3.1 Brain Swelling and Cerebral Edema

Swelling of the brain is a frequent adverse of TBI and represents a leading cause of morbidity and mortality in severely head-injured patients [4]. Swelling most often represents the macroscopic correlate for cerebral edema although may uncommonly develop as a consequence of cerebral hyperemia.

Cerebral edema is defined by an increased water content of the brain, which may be affect the extracellular space, vasogenic edema, or be the consequence of alterations of cellular homeostasis leading to cytotoxic edema. Vasogenic edema, often considered as the most common form of posttraumatic edema, represents the consequence of structural and functional alterations of the blood-brain barrier leading to a shift of fluid from cerebral vessels into the extracellular space. Cytotoxic edema develops shortly after the injury as the consequence of membrane depolarization leading to a generalized release of glutamate causing the activation of N-methyl-D-aspartate and α-amino-3-hydroxy-5-methyl-4-isoxazolepropionic acid receptor receptors and the subsequent influx of calcium, sodium, and water within the cells [5]. Intracellular calcium accumulation, along with associated noxious signals such as ischemia and oxidative stress, results in progressive mitochondrial damage and energy crisis. As intracellular ATP availability is compromised, energy-dependent ionic pumps fail, and water and accumulating ions cannot be expelled back in the extracellular space.

Cerebral hyperemia is an uncommon situation characterized by impairment of cerebral autoregulation with sudden onset of cerebral blood flow increased mediated by vasodilation leading to cerebral congestion. This condition may be responsible for a fast increase in ICP and occurs mostly in children and young adults. Accurate diagnosis of this relatively rare condition is essential for it requires specific therapeutic measures that may be even detrimental in the presence of cerebral edema.

12.3.2 Cerebral Blood Flow

Impairment of cerebral blood flow (CBF) following severe TBI has been repeatedly reported [6, 7], particularly in the early posttraumatic period. Oligemia due to increased intracranial pressure and impaired autoregulation has been shown to be associated with unfavorable functional outcome, and signs of ischemia can be found in most instances of lethal TBI. Patients with subdural hematoma and diffuse cerebral swelling are more likely to suffer from cerebral ischemia. Furthermore, CBF may be further compromised throughout the course of illness as the consequence of developing brain swelling and cerebral vasospasm mediated by traumatic subarachnoid hemorrhage [8].

12.3.3 Cerebral Metabolism

Depressed cerebral metabolism has been identified as an important physiologic hallmark of TBI, and oxidative metabolism rates as low as half the value found under normal conditions have been reported in several studies [9]. Energy crisis has been commonly attributed to compromised oxygen delivery induced by cerebral ischemia, although spreading cortical depression in comatose and sedated patients is another advocated hypothesis. Recent studies, however, have emphasized the pivotal role played by mitochondrial damage mediated by a vast array of noxious stimuli integrated and amplified within the mitochondrion, in failure of ATP production [10]. Furthermore, recent clinical studies have shown that the level of metabolic depression correlated with the level of consciousness, whereas animal studies showed that mitochondrial protection was associated with both improved metabolism and ICP relief [11].

12.4 Critical Care Management

12.4.1 Intracranial Pressure Monitoring and Control

Elevated ICP has been reported to be an independent predictor of increased mortality and is associated with poor functional outcome. Although ICP levels as low as 15 mmHg may be sufficient to prompt cerebral herniation at particular location, a threshold of 20–25 mmHg is currently considered to justify implementation of therapeutic measures [12]. Accordingly, ICP monitoring should be performed in all severe TBI patients. Absence or delay of ICP monitoring has been recently shown to be associated with increased mortality and worse outcome [13].

12.4.2 Mechanical Ventilation, Analgesics, and Sedations

Mechanical ventilation is commonly initiated at prehospital stage or on admission to the emergency room for airway control in patients with severe TBI. Further, mechanical ventilation is often necessary in patients with impaired consciousness in order to prevent superimposed hypoxemic insults and ICP elevation caused by hypercarbia. Hyperventilation should not be used unless CBF measurements can be obtained and the effect of hypocarbia on cerebral perfusion assessed, especially during the first 24 h of injury and in the presence of cerebral contusions [14, 15]. In severe TBI patients, mechanical ventilation as well as general ICU and nursing procedures may be occasionally painful and generate transient and harmful ICP elevations. For this reason, sedation and analgesics should be liberally implemented in patients' general care, using drugs that can be easily titrated and characterized by rapid onset and offset. Propofol is currently the sedative of choice as its effect can be reversed within a short time whenever indicated and is anticonvulsant as well. Propofol is also an efficient drug for ICP control. Midazolam may be used alternatively, providing a potent anticonvulsive effect with lesser cardiovascular depression. Muscle relaxants should not be used on a routine basis though may be recommended in the presence of refractory intracranial hypertension [16].

12.4.3   Hyperosmolar Therapy

Mannitol is the most commonly used hypo-osmotic agent for reduction of ICP. Its effect is produced by osmotic reduction of the cerebral water content and presumably by a beneficial rheologic effect due to hematocrit reduction and plasma volume increase. The use of mannitol is recommended only in the presence of elevated ICP. Prophylactic use of mannitol is not recommended unless clinical signs of cerebral herniation develop prior initiation of ICP monitoring. Mannitol is contraindicated in the presence of arterial hypertension, serum osmolarity ≥320 m)sm/l, sepsis, and signs of renal failure.

Hypertonic saline represents an alternative to mannitol that has gained recently increasing acceptance. Accumulating evidence has suggested that HS may be more effective than mannitol, even at iso-osmolar doses [17, 18], presumably because of a stronger osmotic power and some additional properties such as significant CBF augmentation and anti-inflammatory properties. In a recent randomized control study, however, HS failed to prove to be more effective than mannitol for ICP control though its cerebral hemodynamic impact did prove to be significantly stronger which may be of importance in the presence of cerebral ischemia [19].

12.4.4 Cerebral Perfusion Pressure Management

Although elevation of cerebral perfusion pressure (CPP) does not necessarily result in a proportionate CBF increase, systemic hypotension and low CPP between 50 mmHg may worsen pre-existing ischemia especially in focal forms of TBI leading to poorer outcome and should be therefore avoided. Several studies have suggested a beneficial effect of CPP elevation above 70 mmHg although the effect of CPP elevation depends on preservation of autoregulation [20]. Under physiological conditions, improvement of cerebral perfusion mediated by CPP elevation results in pH increase in subsequent vasoconstriction and decrease in cerebral blood volume. On the contrary, in the presence of impaired autoregulation, CPP elevation may be responsible for cerebral congestion and even worsen preexisting intracranial hypertension. Furthermore, CPP-targeted therapy aiming at the maintenance of CPP above 70 mmHg was found to be associated with increased risk of ARDS [21], justifying the lowering of the previously recommended CPP threshold down to 60 mmHg.

Thresholds goals should be ideally achieved by vigorous fluid resuscitation, based on isotonic crystalloids and blood products when indicated under monitoring of central venous pressure. Excessive fluid administration should be avoided because of the risk of lung complications and increased rebleeding from peripheral injured blood vessels in uncontrolled hemorrhagic shock [22]. Failure to raise CPP despite appropriate resuscitation should prompt the use of vasopressors. Norepinephrine is the vasopressor of choice in TBI although phenylephrine is a pure alpha-agonist can be conveniently used in TBI patients with tachycardia.

12.4.5 Hypothermia

Despite of solid experimental evidence showing the beneficial effect of hypothermia in TBI, clinical evidence supporting the routine use of prophylactic hypothermia is lacking and its role on neurological outcome is debated. Analysis of published RCTs, however, suggests that maintenance of temperature at 32–33 for 48 h is associated with better odds of good neurological outcome [23]. On the opposite, uncontrolled hyperpyrexia should be avoided and fever aggressively treated in severe TBI patients.

12.4.6 Steroids

In the view of a wealthy bulk of evidence provided by a vast number of experimental studies, the use of steroids in TBI patients seems a logical step forward. However, the CRASH multicenter international trial has shown that the effect of steroids was counterintuitively detrimental in TBI [24] so that steroids are not recommended and that high-dose methylprednisolone is currently contraindicated in this indication of neural injury.

12.5 Acute Head Injuries and Their Surgical Management

12.5.1 Skull Fractures

Linear skull fractures represent the consequent of an impact to the skull with energy applied to a broad area preventing penetration. Linear fractures have little consequences by themselves and do not require any particular treatment though are indicative of significant head injury and may be associated with meningeal vessels injury leading to epidural hematoma.

Depressed fractures are caused by high energy impact or contact load delivered by small hard objects creating a penetrating force through the skull, displacing bone fragments intracranially. Depressed fractures may be simple or complex and comminuted according to the impact characteristics and the site of injury. Depressed fractures are commonly associated with scalp wounds that should be carefully investigated for the presence of lacerated brain tissue and cerebrospinal fluid (CSF) leak. Computerized tomography will allow a thorough evaluation of the fracture, disclosing associated brain lesions such as cerebral contusion and hematomas, intracranial air bubbles often indicative of a dural tear, and involvement of venous sinuses at risk of secondary thrombosis.

Basilar fractures may be the consequence of a direct blow to prominent regions of the head adjacent to the cranial base such as the occiput, the mastoid, and the orbital rim. They may also occur as an extension of fracture lines to the cranial base, originating from either the cranial vault or facial bones. Basilar fractures are often associated with dural tear leading to CSF leak and less often with injuries to cranial nerves and basal cerebral vessels.

12.5.2 Epidural Hematoma

Epidural hematomas (EDHs) usually represent a complication of striping of the dura initiated by skull deformation and are therefore associated with skull fractures in most instances. EDHs are reported in 2–4 % of all TBIs [25]. Their relatively low mortality, less than 10 %, testifies the absence of significant underlying brain pathology in most instances although associated intracranial hemorrhage has been reported with an incidence as high as 30–50 %. Epidural bleeding is commonly caused by injury to dural arteries or veins by the edges of the fracture bone though may arise from injured dural sinuses or veins of the diploe, especially in children. EDHs most often develop in the temporal regions as the consequence of injury to the middle meningeal artery and may expand rapidly causing early neurological deterioration and tentorial herniation if not promptly evacuated.

In most instances, EDHs should be treated surgically, leading to mortality as low as 5–10 %. However, small supratentorial hematomas (volume less than 300 cc, less than 10 mm thick with less than 5 mm midline shift) can be conservatively managed in patients without focal neurological deficit. Even small infratentorial hematomas should be more carefully considered for conservative management as herniation may develop without signs of mass effect. Eventually, up to 50 % of conservatively managed EDHs will show some degree of enlargement leading to neurological deterioration prompting emergency craniotomy in some patients.

12.5.3 Acute Subdural Hematoma

Two different mechanisms may be responsible for acute subdural hematoma (ASDH), leading to two distinct pathological situations. In the first instance, ASDH appears as a complication of brain laceration or contusion caused by impact load. In such situation, a significant brain injury is usually associated with subdural bleeding, accounting for a persistent loss of consciousness and high mortality rates. In the second instance, ASDH develops as the consequence of rupture of bridging veins stretched by acceleration-deceleration injury. In that situation, there is no significant focal injury, and patients may initially present with minimal neurological signs before the rapid onset on secondary deterioration [25].

CT scan equally discloses a crescentic, extra-axial hyperdense mass, typically responsible for a midline shift in excess of hematoma thickness indicative of associated underlying brain edema. Any mass thicker than 10 mm with a midline shift higher than 5 mmHg or causing neurological deterioration and/ or ICP increase should prompt rapid evacuation of the subdural clot. A large craniotomy is preferred for this purpose, especially if decompressive craniectomy is contemplated in the view of the lesions depicted by preoperative CT scan.

Prognosis of ASDH is grim with mortality rates as high as 50–70 %. Although mortality has been closely related to the time elapsed until surgery with a cutoff time of 4 h, several other important factors have shown to affect outcome such as age ≥ 65 associated with 82 % mortality and the neurological status at the time of surgery [25].

12.5.4 Cerebral Contusions and Intracerebral Hematoma

Cerebral contusions represent one of the most common traumatic findings, present in up to 31 % of initial imaging studies [26]. Cerebral contusions may develop at the point of impact (coup contusions) or oppositely as a result of acceleration-deceleration, setting the brain in motion within the skull (contrecoup contusions). Such relative and fast motion of the brain is responsible for surface lesions generated at critical protruding aspects of the skull such as the orbital roof, the sphenoid ridge, and the pole of the middle fossa. Accordingly, most of cerebral contusions are located in the temporal and frontal lobes as a consequence of the brain impacting against the skull. Parietal and occipital lobe hematomas are much less common and are usually due to direct impact. Structurally, cerebral contusions are characterized by an area of hemorrhagic necrosis surrounded by perilesional edema. One of the most distinctive features of cerebral contusions is their capacity to enlarge and become significant space-occupying intracranial lesions, leading to increased intracranial pressure and neurological deterioration. Studies based on serial imaging related this deterioration to evolving edema in the area surrounding the contusion and enlargement of the hemorrhagic component of the lesions [27]. In a series of 729 TBI patients surveyed by the European Brain Injury Consortium, cerebral contusions alone (44 %) or in association with subdural hematoma (29 %) represented the most frequent indication for delayed surgical intervention [28].

As such, cerebral contusions represent a major therapeutic challenge by including a potentially growing mass mixed with presumably viable tissue, which may be of critical functional importance whenever surgical removal of the lesion is contemplated in neurologically eloquent areas. This inhomogeneity is often reflected on the initial computerized tomography (CT) by a salt-and-pepper appearance. Although there is little debate that hyperdense regions represent hemorrhagic areas that can be safely evacuated, the significance of surrounding hypodense regions is a matter of controversies. Even though the decision for removing a hematoma in the absence of neurological worsening or ICP elevation is somehow controversial.

As a rule of the thumb, patients with intracerebral hematoma with signs of progressive neurological deterioration or uncontrolled intracranial hypertension should be managed surgically. Radiological criteria for surgery should include hematomas larger than 50 cc or temporal lesions larger than 20 cc and the presence of mass effect represented by either midline shift larger than 5 mm or compression of basal cisterns [25].

12.5.5 *Brain Swelling and Decompressive Craniectomy*

Emerging from simple physical principles, the concept of decompressive craniectomy (DC) has been advocated since 1894 for control and relief of ICP. Although intuitively appealing and usually effective for ICP control, it is not clear whether or not DC improves neurological outcome. In spite of a broad implementation in the presence of refractory intracranial hypertension, DC proved to positively affect outcome only in pediatric TBI, whereas solid evidence of any beneficial effect of DC in adults is lacking [29]. Several studies, mostly retrospective in nature, have shown that DC resulted in significant ICP decrease. In a recent multicenter randomized trial, however, improved ICP control proved to be associated with an increased proportion of patients with poor functional outcome [30].

Nevertheless, DC remains a sound mean of rescue ICP relief for patients admitted with GCS score higher than 6 and presenting with neurological worsening and at risk of cerebral herniation. Whenever indicated, DC may be performed by either a large hemispheric craniectomy or bifrontal decompression, according to the distribution of TBI lesions and the presence of a midline shift. There is no evidence, however, whether the DC should be performed prophylactically early in the course of the illness or in response to ICP elevation.

References

1. Doppenberg EM, Choi SC, Bullock R (2004) Clinical trials in traumatic brain injury: lessons for the future. J Neurosurg Anesthesiol 16(1):87–94
2. Coronado VG, Xu L (2011) Surveillance for traumatic brain injury-related deaths: United States, 1997–2007. U.S. Department of Health and Human Services, Centers for Disease Control and Prevention, Atlanta, p 32

3. Gennarelli TA (1983) Head injury in man and experimental animals: clinical aspects. Acta Neurochir Suppl (Wien) 32:1–13
4. Treggiari MM, Schutz N, Yanez ND, Romand JA (2007) Role of intracranial pressure values and patterns in predicting outcome in traumatic brain injury: a systematic review. Neurocrit Care 6(2):104–112
5. Simon RP, Griffiths T, Evans MC, Swan JH, Meldrum BS (1984) Calcium overload in selectively vulnerable neurons of the hippocampus during and after ischemia: an electron microscopy study in the rat. J Cereb Blood Flow Metab 4(3):350–361
6. Jaggi JL, Obrist WD, Gennarelli TA, Langfitt TW (1990) Relationship of early cerebral blood flow and metabolism to outcome in acute head injury. J Neurosurg 72(2295915):176–182
7. Robertson CS, Gopinath SP, Goodman JC, Contant CF, Valadka AB, Narayan RK (1995) SjvO2 monitoring in head-injured patients. J Neurotrauma 12(5):891–896
8. Martin NA, Patwardhan RV, Alexander MJ, Africk CZ, Lee JH, Shalmon E, Hovda DA, Becker DP (1997) Characterization of cerebral hemodynamic phases following severe head trauma: hypoperfusion, hyperemia, and vasospasm. J Neurosurg 87(9202259):9–19
9. Soustiel JF, Glenn TC, Shik V, Boscardin J, Mahamid E, Zaaroor M (2005) Monitoring of cerebral blood flow and metabolism in traumatic brain injury. J Neurotrauma 22(9):955–965
10. Vespa P, Bergsneider M, Hattori N, Wu HM, Huang SC, Martin NA, Glenn TC, McArthur DL, Hovda DA (2005) Metabolic crisis without brain ischemia is common after traumatic brain injury: a combined microdialysis and positron emission tomography study. J Cereb Blood Flow Metab 25(6):763–774
11. Soustiel JF, Vlodavsky E, Milman F, Gavish M, Zaaroor M (2011) Improvement of cerebral metabolism mediated by Ro5-4864 is associated with relief of intracranial pressure and mitochondrial protective effect in experimental brain injury. Pharm Res 28(11):2945–2953
12. Bratton SL, Chestnut RM, Ghajar J, McConnell Hammond FF, Harris OA, Hartl R, Manley GT, Nemecek A, Newell DW, Rosenthal G, Schouten J, Shutter L, Timmons SD, Ullman JS, Videtta W, Wilberger JE, Wright DW (2007) Guidelines for the management of severe traumatic brain injury. VIII. Intracranial pressure thresholds. J Neurotrauma 24 Suppl 1:S55–S58
13. Barmparas G, Singer M, Ley E, Chung R, Malinoski D, Margulies D, Salim A, Bukur M (2012) Decreased intracranial pressure monitor use at level II trauma centers is associated with increased mortality. Am Surg 78(10):1166–1171
14. Coles JP, Minhas PS, Fryer TD, Smielewski P, Aigbirihio F, Donovan T, Downey SP, Williams G, Chatfield D, Matthews JC, Gupta AK,

Carpenter TA, Clark JC, Pickard JD, Menon DK (2002) Effect of hyperventilation on cerebral blood flow in traumatic head injury: clinical relevance and monitoring correlates. Crit Care Med 30(9): 1950–1959

15. Muizelaar JP, Marmarou A, Ward JD, Kontos HA, Choi SC, Becker DP, Gruemer H, Young HF (1991) Adverse effects of prolonged hyperventilation in patients with severe head injury: a randomized clinical trial. J Neurosurg 75(5):731–739

16. Haddad SH, Arabi YM (2012) Critical care management of severe traumatic brain injury in adults. Scand J Trauma Resusc Emerg Med 20:12

17. Kamel H, Navi BB, Nakagawa K, Hemphill JC 3rd, Ko NU (2011) Hypertonic saline versus mannitol for the treatment of elevated intracranial pressure: a meta-analysis of randomized clinical trials. Crit Care Med 39(3):554–559

18. Oddo M, Levine JM, Frangos S, Carrera E, Maloney-Wilensky E, Pascual JL, Kofke WA, Mayer SA, LeRoux PD (2009) Effect of mannitol and hypertonic saline on cerebral oxygenation in patients with severe traumatic brain injury and refractory intracranial hypertension. J Neurol Neurosurg Psychiatry 80(8):916–920

19. Cottenceau V, Masson F, Mahamid E, Petit L, Shik V, Sztark F, Zaaroor M, Soustiel JF (2011) Comparison of effects of equiosmolar doses of mannitol and hypertonic saline on cerebral blood flow and metabolism in traumatic brain injury. J Neurotrauma 28(10): 2003–2012

20. Rosner MJ, Daughton S (1990) Cerebral perfusion pressure management in head injury. J Trauma 30(8):933–940; discussion 940–941

21. Robertson CS, Valadka AB, Hannay HJ, Contant CF, Gopinath SP, Cormio M, Uzura M, Grossman RG (1999) Prevention of secondary ischemic insults after severe head injury. Crit Care Med 27(10): 2086–2095

22. Solomonov E, Hirsh M, Yahiya A, Krausz MM (2000) The effect of vigorous fluid resuscitation in uncontrolled hemorrhagic shock after massive splenic injury. Crit Care Med 28(3):749–754

23. Henderson WR, Dhingra VK, Chittock DR, Fenwick JC, Ronco JJ (2003) Hypothermia in the management of traumatic brain injury. A systematic review and meta-analysis. Intensive Care Med 29(10): 1637–1644

24. Roberts I, Yates D, Sandercock P, Farrell B, Wasserberg J, Lomas G, Cottingham R, Svoboda P, Brayley N, Mazairac G, Laloe V, Munoz-Sanchez A, Arango M, Hartzenberg B, Khamis H, Yutthakasemsunt S, Komolafe E, Olldashi F, Yadav Y, Murillo-Cabezas F, Shakur H,

Edwards P (2004) Effect of intravenous corticosteroids on death within 14 days in 10008 adults with clinically significant head injury (MRC CRASH trial): randomised placebo-controlled trial. Lancet 364(9442): 1321–1328

25. Zacko JC, Harris L, Bullock MR (2011) Surgical management of traumatic brain injury. In: Win HR (ed) Youmans neurological surgery, vol 4. Elsevier Saunders, Philadelphia, pp 3424–3452
26. Lobato RD, Cordobes F, Rivas JJ, de la Fuente M, Montero A, Barcena A, Perez C, Cabrera A, Lamas E (1983) Outcome from severe head injury related to the type of intracranial lesion. A computerized tomography study. J Neurosurg 59(5):762–774
27. Servadei F, Nanni A, Nasi MT, Zappi D, Vergoni G, Giuliani G, Arista A (1995) Evolving brain lesions in the first 12 hours after head injury: analysis of 37 comatose patients. Neurosurgery 37(5):899–906; discussion 906–907
28. Compagnone C, Murray GD, Teasdale GM, Maas AI, Esposito D, Princi P, D'Avella D, Servadei F (2005) The management of patients with intradural post-traumatic mass lesions: a multicenter survey of current approaches to surgical management in 729 patients coordinated by the European Brain Injury Consortium. Neurosurgery 57(6): 1183–1192; discussion 1183–1192
29. Sahuquillo J, Arikan F (2006) Decompressive craniectomy for the treatment of refractory high intracranial pressure in traumatic brain injury. Cochrane Database Syst Rev (1):CD003983
30. Cooper DJ, Rosenfeld JV, Murray L, Arabi YM, Davies AR, D'Urso P, Kossmann T, Ponsford J, Seppelt I, Reilly P, Wolfe R (2011) Decompressive craniectomy in diffuse traumatic brain injury. N Engl J Med 364(16):1493–1502

Chapter 13
Establishing a Trauma Service

David J.J. Muckart and Noel Naidoo

Trauma has rightly been referred to as an epidemic [1, 2], the definition of which is "a condition affecting many people in any one region at the same time." On a global scale injury is the commonest cause of death under the age of 45 years and accounts for more years of life lost than any other disease process. The fiscal burden goes far beyond the outlay required to manage trauma, for those most affected are the young productive members of society on whom much has been spent in education and training for ultimately no return on investment. Any other disease process which culls the youth to such an extent would result in a national outcry, but for inexplicable reasons governments have been slow to react despite the evidence. For that reason political will is the first essential step when establishing a trauma service for it is an expensive business to run, and the financial benefits will not be evident for at least a decade. Does it justify the capital outlay? All countries which

D.J.J. Muckart, FRCS, MMedSci (✉) • N. Naidoo, FCS (SA)
Department of Surgery, Nelson R Mandela School of Medicine,
University of KwaZulu-Natal, 719 Umbilo Road,
Durban, Republic of South Africa
e-mail: davidmuc@ialch.co.za; noel.naidoo@gmail.com

S. Di Saverio et al. (eds.), *Trauma Surgery*,
DOI 10.1007/978-88-470-5403-5_13, © Springer-Verlag Italia 2014

have invested in dedicated trauma services have shown marked improvements in resuscitation, timing of surgical intervention, survival, and reductions in preventable deaths [3–5].

A trauma service should be viewed as a continuum of care beginning with the prehospital care providers and ending with rehabilitation and a return to productivity. In the midst are various levels of trauma care with specific designations depending on verification status [6]. To establish an efficient service, each and every aspect must be addressed. It is an exercise in futility establishing a sophisticated prehospital service which has no appropriate destination or constructing Trauma Units to the highest architectural and equipment standards which have no delivery service or cannot be staffed with experienced personnel.

13.1 Prehospital Care [7]

All levels of prehospital care, whether at basic, intermediate, or advanced levels of support, are integral to an effective trauma system. Prompt care by well-trained personnel reduces the incidence of early and delayed deaths. Although advanced life support is undoubtedly effective and attractive, the benefit applies to the least number of trauma patients, and appropriate number of crews trained in intermediate life support would have a greater overall effect on improved survival. The triage adage of saving the maximum number of lives applies.

There are certain key elements to a successful prehospital service. There must be support at the highest government level to ensure finance and legislation governing the authority to run a prehospital service, training, scope of practice, licensure, and accreditation. At both national and regional levels, whether the service is governmental or private, leadership is essential for implementation and ensuring adherence to national legislation and standards. A Medical Director with experience or accreditation in Accident and Emergency Medicine or an allied discipline must be appointed to facilitate recruitment and training, supervise continuing education, develop standard operating procedures, and ensure adherence to national legislation.

In addition to ground transfer vehicles, aeromedical capability, both helicopter and fixed wing need to be considered. The type and number will be dictated by demand, terrain, time, and distance to definitive care. Although air transfer is rapid, the costs of maintaining such a service are substantial, and the need must be justified and strict criteria in place to ensure optimal use.

The decision to transport patients to a Level I center based on observations in the field can be difficult. Criteria for Level I referral are based on four parameters, namely, extremes of age, physiological instability, mechanism of injury, and existing comorbidities. The Revised Trauma Score [8] which provides an objective estimate of severity based on the Glasgow Coma Scale, systolic blood pressure, and respiratory rate is the most commonly used method, and an overtriage rate of 10–15 % is the accepted norm.

13.2 Hospital Designation [6]

In the middle of the trauma service is the lead hospital or major trauma center, the Level I tertiary facility capable of providing all necessary surgery and the highest level of ICU support. Such a center will be affiliated to a university and must be involved in trauma prevention, education, research, and system planning and be the lead hospital for a regional trauma service. Level II or regional centers should be capable of providing advanced life support and any necessary life-saving surgery but may not possess all the necessary surgical disciplines or ICU capabilities. A Level III or district center must be capable of initial advanced life support if necessary, but thereafter transfer will be required for definitive care. Level IV facilities are primary health-care facilities which may vary in capability but should be integrated into a trauma network. All patients who require the resources of a Level I center should have access to it regardless of the level of initial care facility, and any level of initial care must be capable of direct referral to the highest level without progression through intermediate health institutions.

The required number of the specific levels of care will be dictated by population density and need based on trauma epidemiology. There is little benefit to be gained from establishing Level I centers in areas with a low trauma prevalence. This not only is cost ineffective but dilutes exposure and experience, and the need would be better served by regional institutions without having a major effect on outcome as long as an efficient prehospital service is in place for rapid transportation to a Level I facility. Conversely, there may be a need for more than one Level I center in high-density urban developments.

13.3 Hospital Accreditation for a Level I Center [6]

13.3.1 Patient Profile

Major trauma centers should manage an average of 1,200 patients per year of which at least 20 % should have an Injury Severity Score (ISS) of 15 or greater *or* there should be 35 patients per surgeon with an ISS > 15.

13.3.2 Staffing

Essential to a Level I service is the 24-h in-house availability of a general surgeon, orthopedic surgeon, and anesthetist. Supervising these must be a general surgeon accredited in trauma and with experience in critical care, whose responsibility is to coordinate all aspects of care from initial resuscitation to discharge. Although not necessarily in-house for a 24-h period, the senior surgeon's attendance at all admissions, resuscitations, and emergency operative procedures is mandatory. Immediately available must be the subspecialties of neurosurgery, plastic surgery, cardiothoracic surgery, and pediatric surgery although in certain countries the senior trauma surgeon may have enough operative expertise in some of these disciplines. Allied healthcare personnel such as psychologists, physiotherapists, occupational therapists, critical care technologists, and nursing staff trained in emergency medicine and critical care are equally essential.

13.3.3   Unit Architecture

The location of the major trauma center within the hospital should allow rapid, direct, and unobstructed access for both road and air transfer. As far as possible the unit should be self-sufficient, incorporating a mass casualty receiving area for disaster management with each bay being serviced by enough piped oxygen, medical air, vacuum, and electrical points to provide care equivalent to basic ICU standards. Ceiling-mounted supply pods are preferred in this area and any individual resuscitation rooms as they permit unobstructed access to the patient, whereas floor-mounted service pods are acceptable within the ICU where interventions are rather more controlled. Dedicated resuscitation rooms should be equipped to ICU standards and contain moveable overhead lights as within the operating theater. One resuscitation room should be dedicated to pediatrics and equipped as such.

There must be a dedicated trauma theater within the unit [9], the operating table allowing radiological imaging for fracture management. To prevent the need for changing operating tables, ideally two theaters should be commissioned, one for major fracture management and the other for general procedures. In view of the potential urgency for operative intervention, it is unacceptable for trauma patients to share operative facilities with other disciplines.

A point of care laboratory must contain a blood gas analyzer with electrolyte and lactate analysis and thromboelastography. Standard electrolyte, liver function, and coagulation testing will be undertaken by a central laboratory. The hospital must contain a blood bank and the unit a fridge for storing at least two units of O negative blood.

A dedicated ultrasound machine within the resuscitation room is essential for FAST scanning. Designed in South Africa, low-density x-ray screening (LODOX) has become popular and proved exceptionally accurate for initial screening [10], although CT angiography is required for multiply injured patients. Due to expense it may be impractical to house a dedicated scanner within the unit, but access must be immediate to a common scanner and the radiology department located in close proximity on the same floor.

13.3.4 Intensive Care

Paradoxically the nomenclature for ICU classification is the converse of Trauma Units with a Level III ICU providing all interventions necessary for support of organ system failure and Level I offering high dependency only. In between lies a Level II unit which may provide initial invasive mechanical ventilation and hemodynamic support but cannot undertake renal replacement therapy (RRT) or more specialized interventions for organ dysfunction. The major trauma center must contain a

Level III ICU, regional trauma hospitals (Level II) should be capable of providing basic intensive care, but Level III trauma facilities will not be required or able to offer any support above high dependency, and even then, such patients would be better managed in a higher facility. The Level I Trauma Unit should encompass a dedicated Level III intensive care unit which functions on a closed basis. All management decisions should be the responsibility of the senior trauma surgeon and colleagues and not deferred to subspecialists in other disciplines. Mortality and morbidity rates are higher in ICUs which function on an open basis [11]. The needs of the critically injured are not the same as non-trauma patients, and housing trauma patients in a surgical or mixed medical-surgical intensive care unit is best avoided.

13.3.5 Protocols and Audit

Although each patient must be managed on an individual basis, protocols must be in place as general guidelines for admission and discharge, resuscitation, the need for damage control, sedation and analgesia, enteral and parenteral feeding, venous thrombosis prophylaxis, glycemic control, stress ulcer prophylaxis, infection control, and antimicrobial use.

Audit and an assessment of morbidity and mortality are essential to compare outcomes with national and international norms and identify areas for improvement, research publications, and system planning. Prevention is far cheaper and more effective than cure, and a trauma system should include public education and awareness programs and recommendations to legislative bodies concerning the need for any changes in the law which may reduce the prevalence of injury.

References

1. Baker SP (1987) Injuries: the neglected epidemic. J Trauma 27: 343–348
2. Muckart DJJ (1991) Trauma – the malignant epidemic. S Afr J Med 79:93–95
3. West JG, Cales RH, Gazzaniga AB (1983) Impact of regionalisation. The Orange County experience. Arch Surg 118:740–744
4. Celso B, Tepas J, Langland-Orban B et al (2006) A systematic review and meta-analysis comparing outcome of severely injured patients treated in trauma centers following the establishment of trauma systems. J Trauma 60:371–378
5. Rotondo MF, Bard MR, Sagraves SG et al (2009) What price commitment: what benefit? The cost of a saved life in a developing level I trauma center. J Trauma 67:915–923
6. Committee on Trauma American College of Surgeons (1998) Resources for optimal care of the injured patient 1999. The American College of Surgeons, Chicago
7. Sasser S, Varghese M, Kellerman A et al (2005) Prehospital trauma care systems. World Health Organisation Press, WHO Geneva
8. Champion HR, Sacco WJ, Copes WS et al (1989) A revision of the Trauma Score. J Trauma 29:623–629
9. Brasel KJ, Akanson J, Weigelt JA (1998) The dedicated operating room for trauma: a costly recommendation. J Trauma 14:832–838
10. Chen RJ, Fu CY, Wu SC et al (2010) Diagnostic accuracy, biohazard safety, and cost effectiveness-the Lodox/Statscan provides a beneficial alternative for the primary evaluation of patients with multiple injuries. J Trauma 69:826–830
11. Treggiari MM, Martin DP, Yanez ND et al (2007) Effect of intensive care unit organizational model and structure on outcomes in patients with acute lung injury. Am J Respir Crit Care Med 176:685–690

Chapter 14
Multiple Organ Failure in Trauma Patients

Francesco Del Corso, Carlo Coniglio, Aimone Giugni, Francesca Mengoli, Francesco Boni, Ilaria Turriziani, Gregorio Tugnoli, Salomone Di Saverio, and Giovanni Gordini

14.1 Introduction

Progress in resuscitation, damage control, and critical care techniques in the last 50 years have decreased mortality of trauma patients, enabling severely ill patient to survive the early phase of injury but resulting in subsequent dysfunction or failure of several organs function called multiple organ failure (MOF) syndrome. Postinjury MOF is in general secondary to massive systemic inflammatory syndrome that occurs after the traumatic event, and if traditionally was defined as the occurrence of two or

F. Del Corso • C. Coniglio (✉) • A. Giugni • F. Mengoli • F. Boni
I. Turriziani • G. Gordini
Department of Emergency, Intensive Care Unit-HEMS,
Maggiore Hospital, Largo Bartolo Nigrisoli 2, Bologna 40100, Italy
e-mail: delcorsofrancesco@gmail.com; car.coniglio@gmail.com;
aimonegiugni@gmail.com; f.mengoli@118er.it; boni.doc@gmail.com;
ilariaturriz@gmail.com; g.gordini@118er.it

G. Tugnoli • S. Di Saverio
Trauma Surgery Unit, Maggiore Hospital Regional Trauma Center,
Largo Bartolo Nigrisoli 2, AUSL Bologna 40100, Bologna, Italy
e-mail: gregorio.tugnoli@ausl.bologna.it; salo75@inwind.it

S. Di Saverio et al. (eds.), *Trauma Surgery*,
DOI 10.1007/978-88-470-5403-5_14, © Springer-Verlag Italia 2014

more organ failures, over the years from the original all-or-none concept, it moved into a dynamic definition of this syndrome as a continuous process of varying levels of organ dysfunction.

Over the last 50 years, mortality associated with this syndrome is decreased but still remains the most significant cause (51–61 %) of late trauma death [1, 2].

14.2 Definitions

The trauma, causing blood loss, hypotension, hypoperfusion and major tissue damage, generates immune and inflammatory body responses, both local and systemic, provoked by releasing of proinflammatory cytokines, phospholipids, activation of leukocytes, complements, and all the factors involved in the complex network of the defence host response.

Hyperinflammation – SIRS (*systemic inflammatory response syndrome*) consists of inflammation that involves all the districts of the organism.

SIRS is defined, from 1992 [3], as the presence of two or more of the following criteria:

- Temperature <36° or >38°
- Heart rate >90 bpm/min
- Respiratory rate >20/min or PCO_2 <32 mmHg
- WBC <4,000/ml or >12,000/ml

Hypoinflammation: *CARS* (*Compensatory Anti-inflammatory Response Syndrome*) – Over the same period, or only after a few hours, during which begins the SIRS, the human organism enacts a kind of compensatory response to systemic inflammation, increasing the levels of anti-inflammatory cytokines in the blood, such as IL-10, trying to avoid tissue damage, and consequently minimizing the effects of SIRS. This may explain in part the depletion phase of WBC and lymphocytes that follows trauma. All that is, on the other hand, a double-edged sword because reducing the activity of the immune system is to create a window, a weakness, a perfect gateway for infection and sepsis which increased the risk of MOF [4].

MARS – Mixed antagonistic response syndrome [5] is a hypothetical fight between SIRS and CARS. The human body tries to find a fine balance between tissue damage resulting from inflammation and the risk of infections and susceptibility of the entire system resulting from the reduction of the immune system.

MOF, *Multiple Organ Failure* – As we previously said this syndrome is defined by the simultaneous presence of physiologic dysfunction and/or failure of two or more organs.

Even now there is no consensus on the diagnostic criteria for this syndrome, and in attempting to define it, multiple scoring systems have been used like Denver Postinjury Multiple Organ Failure score, Knaus MOF score, SOFA score, or Marshall score (Tables 14.1 and 14.2).

We can identify two types of MOF depending on the time of onset:

- Early MOF which is a multiple organ failure present at day 3 postinjury.
- Late MOF (60 % of all MOF) [6, 7], a new onset of MOF present after day 3 [4]. The real MOF is a different entity to multiple organ dysfunction syndrome (MODS) that is very common during resuscitation.

14.3 Epidemiology

The mortality of MOF in traumatic patients continues to decline in the course of the years, thanks to the progress made by treatment strategy and new approaches in intensive care unit. In the

Table 14.1 Denver Postinjury Multiple Organ Failure score

Dysfunction	Grade 0	Grade 1	Grade 2	Grade 3
Pulmonary PaO_2/FiO_2	>250	250–200	200–100	<100
Renal creatinine (mg/dl)	<1.8	1.8–2.5	2.5–5.0	>5
Hepatic total bilirubin (mgdl/l)	<2	2–4	4–8	>8
Cardiac	No inotropes	Only 1 inotrope at small dose	Any inotrope at moderate dose or >1 agent at small dose	Any inotrope at large dose or >2 agent at moderate doses

Dewar et al. [4] and Sauaia et al. [29]

The MOF daily score is the addition of the worst values for the day for each organ system. MOF is defined as a score >3

Table 14.2 SOFA score

	Grade 0	Grade 1	Grade 2	Grade 3	Grade 4
Respiratory PaO_2/ FiO_2	>400	<400	<300	<20 with respiratory support	<100 with respiratory support
Coagulation platelets ($\times 10^3$/mm^3)	>150	<150	<100	<50	<20
Liver – bilirubin (mg/dl)	<1.2	1.2–1.9	2.0–5.9	6–11.9	>12
Cardiovascular (vasopressor in mcg/kg/min)	No hypotension	MAP <70 mmHg	Dopamine <= 5 or dobutamine (any dose)	dopamine >5 OR epi <= 0.1 OR nor epi <= 0.1	dop >15 OR epi >0.1 OR nor epi >0.1
Renal – creatinine (mg/dl)	<1.2	1.2–1.9	2.0–3.4	3.5–4.9	>5
CNS – GCS	15	13–14	10–12	6–9	<6

Dewar et al. [4] and Ferreira et al. [30]

MOF is defined as a score of ≥4 with involvement of ≥2 organ systems early 1980s the mortality rate was about 60–100 % [8]; today patients who get postinjury MOF have a mortality rate of 27–100 % depending on the number of organs involved [4].

The incidence of the syndrome instead shows an increase, from the first studies of the 1980s to those of the 1990s, from about 7 to 15 % and remains the same even today [6, 8–10].

Probably this is due to the better understanding of the syndrome and consequently greater ability to recognize and differentiate it.

The most important determinants of MOF's incidence and mortality are factors such as the type and gravity of trauma; different sex, age, and comorbidities; and number of patients who required massive blood transfusion.

The incidence and mortality of single organ failures are also decreased significantly over the years from 22 to 7 % and from 30 to 11 %, respectively [6, 8–10]. The organs affected, however, remain the same, even with the same frequency of interest: lung failure, which usually precedes the cardiac dysfunction of 0.6 days, followed by the liver (4.8 days) and finally by the kidney (5.5 days) [11].

The MOF syndrome is difficult to handle even by the most experienced and remains a major cause of ICU resource use and late mortality after injury.

14.4   Etiology

As previously mentioned, the etiology of the MOF is varied and complex and depends on both the *factors related to the patient* – age, sex, BMI, comorbidities, and genetic predisposition – and the *characteristics of different types of trauma*: severity, ISS, contamination of wounds, and time from injury to treatment.

According to the "second-hit theory," the concept that underlies the onset of the MOF syndrome is the existence of an event

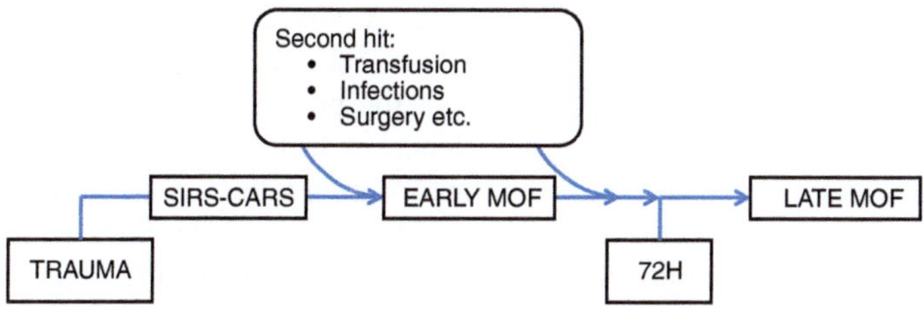

Fig. 14.1 Timing of impending MOF

that acts as first injury, the "first hit," determinating a proinflammatory reaction. It depends on:

- The local damage to tissues and systemic inflammation
- The systemic hypoperfusion following hypotension and oxygenation impairment
- The reperfusion injury which follows the initial successful management

Subsequently an event, such as lung infections, prolonged shock, excessive volume of crystalloid infusions, units of red blood cells, surgery, mechanical ventilation, fat embolism, compartment syndrome, and sepsis, acts as a "second hit," resulting in an uncontrolled inflammation, usually starting during the "vulnerable window" (neutrophilia that occurs early after the traumatic event) [4, 12] and developing the early SIRS in organ failure (Fig. 14.1).

14.5 Pathophysiology

After the trauma, many proinflammatory cytokines, such as IL-1b, IL-6, TNFa, IL-8, IL-12, IL-18, G-CSF, GM-CSF, are immediately released into the circulation that will activate PMNs but also a variety of anti-inflammatory cytokines, for example, IL-1Ra, IL-4, IL-10, IL-11 and IL-13. Usually in homeostasis conditions both sides are balanced and the result is equilibrium. The predominance of the proinflammatory phase leads to SIRS, while the prevalence or lack of control of the inflammatory phase leads to immunosuppression. As mentioned before, a second hit during the CARS or the "vulnerable window," such as an infection, a massive blood transfusion, surgery, respiratory distress with hypoxia, repeated cardiovascular instability, acidosis, and missed injuries, triggers the MOF [13–15].

Some recent studies [16, 17] have shown that in polytrauma patient there are elevated levels of cytokines as TNFs and IL-6 proportionally to the severity of the trauma, confirming the role of this interleukin as a marker of the severity of trauma and as a useful parameter to try to predict the onset of MOF.

TNF-alpha is a cytokine involved in inflammation and stimulates the acute phase reaction; its primary role is in the regulation of immune response. It stimulates the production of NO and activates the cyclooxygenase, promoting the production of thromboxane, prostaglandins, and PAF, unbalancing the endothelial system on behalf the procoagulant factors. TNF-alpha also increases capillary permeability, promoting the migration of neutrophils into the tissue.

The IL-6 is another important cytokine in the genesis of SIRS in trauma; it regulates inflammation; generates C-reactive protein, procalcitonin and fibrinogen; and activates lymphocytes and NK cells. In the genesis of MOF in injured patients, the IL-6 confirms its dual role as both proinflammatory and anti-inflammatory.

The IL-10 is one of most important anti-inflammatory cytokine; its role is exactly the opposite that of the abovementioned cytokines, for example, inhibits the production of monocytes/ macrophages and reduces the proinflammatory mediators.

The complement system plays a key role in the genesis of inflammation after trauma. Sharma et al., Hecke et al., and Kapur et al. have shown that the plasma levels of proinflammatory peptides C3 and C3a increase immediately after trauma [18–20]. The complement cascade causes the formation of pores in cell membranes, resulting in lysis and the production of oxygen free radicals and arachidonic acid metabolites.

In the pathogenesis of MOF are also involved the ischemia/reperfusion injury pathway and the "gut's role."

Ischemia reduces the reserves of ATP, increasing the levels of hypoxanthine and raising intracellular levels of Na^+ and altering those of Ca^{2+}. During the secondary *reperfusion*, the oxygen reacts with hypoxanthine, producing H_2O_2 and the hydroxyl radical $°OH^-$; these reactive oxygen species (ROS, oxygen radicals) contribute to the cell membrane peroxidation, causing diffuse tissue damage.

The splanchnic circulation is the last to be restored after resuscitation [21, 22]. Ischemia and reperfusion may determinate intestinal mucosal barrier dysfunction and bacterial overgrowth, increasing permeability to endotoxins with reduction in immune defense capabilities. This phenomena called bacteria translocation may allow gut-derived toxins and inflammatory mediators to pass the intestinal lymphatic barrier and to reach the systemic circulation, leading to SIRS, ARDS, and MOF [20, 22].

14.6   Clinical Presentation

The clinical entity of MOF presentation depends on the number and severity of the many risk factors responsible of the processes of hypoperfusion, ischemia, and reperfusion which characterize this syndrome [1, 4, 23] (Table 14.3).

Some studies show that males have higher levels of circulating IL-6 after trauma and estrogens may even have a protective role in the development of MOF [4, 24, 25].

The first organ that usually shows signs of malfunction (ARDS, infection) is the lung, followed by heart, liver, and

Table 14.3 Risk factor for developing of MOF

Severity of injury (NISS, ISS > 25)
Units of RBC transfusion greater than 6 within 12 h
Age greater than 55 years
Base deficit greater than 8 mEq at 10–12 h
Lactate levels greater than 2.5 at 12–24 h
Age of transfused blood
Obesity
Abdominal compartment syndrome
Male gender

Dewar D. et al [4]

lastly kidneys [11]. *Lungs* are considered the pacemaker of MOF, considering that half of the circulation is constantly "filtered" by these organs. The signs and symptoms are those of acute respiratory failure (ALI, ARDS), with impairment in oxygenation and CO_2 removal and need of mechanical ventilation. Pulmonary function may be further worsened by direct complication as evolving lung contusion, infection, and fat embolism due to multiple long bone fracture association.

Circulatory failure is associated with the need of vasopressor for maintaining adequate organ perfusion pressure despite adequate volemia.

Liver failure can be manifested by elevations in liver enzymes and bilirubin, coagulation defects, and inability to excrete toxins such as ammonia, which can aggravate encephalopathy.

Coagulopathy in MOF is caused by deficiencies in coagulation system proteins, including protein C, antithrombin III, and tissue factor inhibitors. It should not be confused with the "early" traumatic coagulopathy [26] that is an endogenous impairment of all components of hemostasis that develops rapidly after injury, which is correlated to and contributes to MOF development.

Kidney failure is manifested by oliguria and increase of serum creatinine and BUN, often due to acute tubular necrosis.

Abdominal compartment syndrome should be monitored with bladder pressure and pronto managed in patient at risk (abdominopelvic trauma, massive fluid resuscitated).

Clinical scores (Denver, SOFA, Tables 14.1 and 14.2) are useful diagnostic tools for early detection, prognostication, and monitoring the effect of therapy on management of this sequential organ failure. The early MOF is much more lethal than the late one. The late MOF needs a second hit to start, usually 72 h after trauma [4].

14.7   Treatment

The treatment of multiple organ failure is generally a support therapy.

Current management principles employed in addressing these goals include the following:

1. Early recognition
2. Early organ function support
3. Early hemodynamic resuscitation
4. Early source control and adequate antibiotic therapy in case of infection or sepsis
5. Continued hemodynamic support
6. Metabolic support

The high incidence of early lung failure may require endotracheal intubation and protective mechanical ventilation (low tidal volume as in patient with ARDS) and monitoring of CO_2 levels, including tracheobronchial aspiration of secretions. Control of pulmonary infections is a very key point, and some cultures of tracheobronchial secretions has to be done, to perform the appropriate antibiotic therapy.

The first step for hemodynamic resuscitation is to control any source of bleeding with a good hemostasis starting from damage control intervention (packing, angiography) up to total care when sign of SIRS and MOF attenuate. The second step for hemostatic resuscitation is to detect and control early trauma-induced coagulopathy (TIC), with high ratio (1:1, 1:2) of fresh-frozen plasma (FFP) to packed red blood cells (PRBC) and platelet. TIC is not primarily a consumptive coagulopathy; it is characterized by dysfibrinogenemia, systemic anticoagulation, impaired platelet function, and hyperfibrinolysis. To guide the early goal management of this coagulopathy, instead of traditional laboratory-based clotting screens (PT, aPTT, fibrinogen), viscoelastic coagulation tests [e.g., ROTEM (TEM Innovations GmbH) and TEG (Medicell Ltd)] should be used [26].

Subsequent assessment of the patient's volume and cardiovascular status will guide the amount of fluid resuscitation. In MOF patient clinical assessment of the response to volume infusion may be difficult, and when proper fluid resuscitation fails to restore hemodynamic stability and tissue perfusion, vasopressor therapy has to be started. Under fluid resuscitation as well fluid overload has to be avoided, so these patients require different grade of invasive hemodynamic monitoring from the static one (CVP, arterial lines, pulmonary artery catheters) to functional hemodynamic monitoring which enables to assess, for instance, preload responsiveness of the patient (volume-based monitoring system, echocardiography) [27].

Renal dysfunction, oliguria, and increase in serum creatinine and BUN should prompt attention to adequacy of circulating blood volume, cardiac output, and blood pressure. Not reversible acute kidney injury is an indication to continuous renal replacement therapy (RRT).

Metabolic and nutritional support has an important role in MOF management. Serum glucose should be kept in normal range with insulin infusion to avoid the detrimental effects of hyperglycemia [28].

MOF and critically ill patients are usually hypercatabolic. Early nutritional support via the enteral route is preferred unless the patient has an ileus or other abnormality; gastroparesis is observed commonly and can be treated with motility agents or placement of a small bowel feeding tube.

References

1. Ciesla DJ, Moore EE, Johnson JL et al (2005) A 12-year prospective study of postinjury multiple organ failure: has anything changed? Arch Surg 140(5):432–438
2. Sauaia A, Moore FA, Moore EE et al (1995) Epidemiology of trauma deaths: a reassessment. J Trauma 38(2):185–193
3. Bone RC, Balk RA, Cerra FB et al (1992) Definitions for sepsis and organ failure and guidelines for the use of innovative therapies in sepsis. The ACCP/SCCM Consensus Conference Committee. American College of Chest Physicians/Society of Critical Care Medicine. Chest 101(6):1644–1655
4. Dewar D et al (2009) Postinjury multiple organ failure. Injury 40(9):912–918
5. Bone RC (1996) Sir Isaac Newton, sepsis, SIRS, and CARS. Crit Care Med 24:1125–1128
6. Moore FA, Sauaia A, Moore EE et al (1996) Postinjury multiple organ failure: a bimodal phenomenon. J Trauma 40(4):501–502
7. Sauaia A, Moore FA, Moore EE et al (1998) Multiple organ failure can be predicted as early as 12 h after injury. J Trauma 45(2):291–301
8. Fry DE, Pearlstein L, Fulton RL, Polk HC (1980) Multiple system organ failure: the role of uncontrolled infection. Arch Surg 115(2):136–140
9. Faist E, Baue AE, Dittmer H, Heberer G (1983) Multiple organ failure in polytrauma patients. J Trauma 23(9):775–787
10. Knaus WA, Draper EA, Wagner DP, Zimmerman JE (1985) Prognosis in acute organ-system failure. Ann Surg 202(6):685–693
11. Ciesla DJ, Moore EE, Johnson JL et al (2005) The role of the lung in postinjury multiple organ failure. Surgery 138(4):749–757
12. Moore EE, Moore FA, Harken AH et al (2005) The two-event construct of postinjury multiple organ failure. Shock 24(Suppl 1):71–74
13. Rose S, Marzi I (1996) Pathophysiology of polytrauma. Zentralbl Chir 121:896–913
14. Rotstein OD (2003) Modeling the two-hit hypothesis for evaluating strategies to prevent organ injury after shock/resuscitation. J Trauma 54(Suppl 5):203–206

15. Keel M et al (2005) Pathophysiology of polytrauma. Injury 36:691–709
16. Biffl WL, Moore EE, Moore FA, Peterson VM (1996) Interleukin-6 in the injured patient. Marker of injury or mediator of inflammation? Ann Surg 224:647–664
17. Pape HC, Tsukamoto T, Kobbe P et al (2007) Assessment of the clinical course with inflammatory parameters. Injury 38:1358–1364
18. Sharma DK, Sarda AK, Bhalla SA et al (2004) The effect of recent trauma on serum complement activation and serum C3 levels correlated with the injury severity score. Indian J Med Microbiol 22:147–152
19. Hecke F, Schmidt U, Kola A et al (1997) Circulating complement proteins in multiple trauma patients—correlation with injury severity, development of sepsis, and outcome. Crit Care Med 25:2015–2024
20. Kapur MM, Jain P, Gidh M (1986) The effect of trauma on serum C3 activation and its correlation with injury severity score in man. J Trauma 26:464–466
21. Offner PJ, Moore EE (2000) Risk factors for MOF and pattern of organ failure following severe trauma. In: Baue AE, Faist E, Fry DE (eds) Multiple organ failure. Springer, New York, pp 30–43
22. Tsukamoto T et al (2010) Current theories on the pathophysiology of multiple organ failure after trauma. Injury 41:21–26
23. Sauaia A, Moore FA, Moore EE et al (1994) Early predictors of postinjury multiple organ failure. Arch Surg 129(1):39–45
24. Sperry JL, Friese RS, Frankel HL et al (2007) Male gender is associated with excessiveIL-6 expression following severe injury. J Trauma 63(3):487–493
25. Frink M, Pape HC, van Griensven M et al (2007) Influence of sex and age on mods and cytokines after multiple injuries. Shock 27(2):151–156
26. Frith D, Davenport R, Brohi K (2012) Acute traumatic coagulopathy. Curr Opin Anaesthesiol 25(2):229–234
27. Pinsky M, Payen D (2005) Functional hemodynamic monitoring. Crit Care 9:566–572. doi:10.1186/cc3927
28. Dellinger RP, Levy MM, Carlet JM et al (2008) Surviving Sepsis Campaign: international guidelines for management of severe sepsis and septic shock: 2008. Intensive Care Med 34(1):17–60
29. Sauaia A, Moore EE, Johnson JL, Ciesla DJ, Biffl WL, Banerjee A (2009) Validation of postinjury multiple organ failure scores. Shock 31(5):438–447
30. Ferreira FL, Bota DP, Bross A, Mélot C, Vincent JL (2001) Serial evaluation of the SOFA score to predict outcome in critically ill patients. JAMA 286(14):1754–1758

Chapter 15
Infections in Trauma Patients

Massimo Sartelli and Cristian Tranà

15.1 Introduction

Trauma patients with hospital-acquired infections (HAIs) are at increased risk for mortality, have longer length of stay, and incur higher inpatient costs [1].

Given the magnitude of the clinical and economic burden of HAIs, implementing interventions aiming to decrease the incidence of HAIs may have a potentially very large impact [2].

15.2 Risk Factors

It is well known that patients with traumatic injuries are at increased risk for infection.

The interruption of tissue integrity, hemorrhage and tissue hypoperfusion, frequency of invasive procedures, and impaired

M. Sartelli (⊠) • C. Tranà
Department of Surgery, Hospital of Macerata, Via Santa Lucia, 2,
Macerata 62100, Italy
e-mail: m.sartelli@virgilio.it; cristian.trana@libero.it

S. Di Saverio et al. (eds.), *Trauma Surgery*,
DOI 10.1007/978-88-470-5403-5_15, © Springer-Verlag Italia 2014

host defense mechanisms all have a major impact on subsequent infection [3].

Several factors are implicated in the increased susceptibility of trauma patients to infection, especially in intensive care units (ICU), but identifying independent risk factors for infection in trauma patients is a very difficult task. High ISS scores [4], morbid obesity [5], early hyperglycemia (glucose ≥ 200 mg/dL) [6], the presence of shock or hypoperfusion [7], older age, male gender [8, 9], type of trauma (blunt or penetrating), the number of affected organs, unconsciousness, prolonged mechanical ventilation, spinal cord injury, the requirement for mechanical ventilation, the use of central catheters, multiple transfusions, and several surgical procedures have been reported to be substantial risk factors for infection in trauma patients.

15.3 Pneumonias

Pneumonia is one of the most common hospital-acquired infections in trauma patients.

Injuries to the thorax, head, and abdomen are associated with a significantly increased risk of pneumonia because of changes in respiratory mechanics [10].

However, the main risk factors for hospital-acquired pneumonias (HAPs) in trauma patients are the use of prolonged mechanical ventilation and positive end-expiratory pressure [11].

Ventilator-associated pneumonias (VAPs) are defined as hospital-acquired pneumonias occurring more than 48 h after patients have been intubated and received mechanical ventilation. VAPs are independently associated with death in less severely injured trauma patients [12].

Early pneumonias within the first few days of hospitalization can also result from aspiration at the time of injury.

HAPs are caused by a wide variety of bacteria that originate from the patient flora or the health-care environment. The most commonly isolated organisms are *Staphylococcus aureus*, *Pseudomonas aeruginosa*, *Klebsiella species*, *Escherichia coli*, *Acinetobacter species*, and *Enterobacter species* [13].

Early and appropriate antimicrobial therapy is an essential determinant of clinical outcome. Choosing the appropriate agent, however, remains challenging since in most cases no data on the identity and susceptibility of the pathogen is available at the time of treatment initiation. Because inadequate therapy has been associated with excess hospital mortality from HAPs, the prompt administration of empirical broad-spectrum antimicrobial therapy is essential [14].

15.4 Empyemas

Empyemas after trauma can develop after hemothorax, penetrating trauma to the chest, perforation of the diaphragm, contiguous infection, and prolonged chest tube placement.

Empyema is a rare complication. Gram-positive bacteria are the most likely cause after hemothorax.

Prophylactic antibiotics may be administered at the time of chest tube insertion, though this practice is not routinely recommended.

15.5 Urinary Tract Infections

The development of urinary tract infections (UTIs) is mainly related to indwelling urinary catheter use.

These infections are associated with a greater mortality in trauma patients [15].

Escherichia coli is the most frequent species isolated, although it comprises fewer than one-third of isolates. Other Enterobacteriaceae, such as *Klebsiella* species, *Serratia* species, *Citrobacter* species, and *Enterobacter* species; nonfermenters such as *P. aeruginosa*; and gram-positive cocci, including coagulase-negative staphylococci and *Enterococcus* species, are also isolated.

Use of the urinary catheter should always be discontinued as soon as appropriate. A 7–14-day regimen is recommended for most patients with UTI, regardless whether the patient remains catheterized or not.

Data on local antimicrobial resistance, when available, should be used to help guide empirical treatment. Shorter durations of treatment are preferred in appropriate patients to limit development of resistance. Regimens should be adjusted as appropriate depending on the culture and susceptibility results and the clinical course [16].

15.6 Bloodstream Infections

Resuscitation intravenous lines are a critical part of the care of the trauma patient.

Unfortunately, they are a major source of bloodstream infections.

Central line-associated bloodstream infections (CLABSIs) in critically ill trauma patients are potentially fatal infections and are associated with a substantial increase in long hospital stay and total hospital cost.

Strict adherence to sterile technique can reduce central line-associated bloodstream infections (CLBSIs) and has become a quality improvement measure.

Trauma patients are at higher risk for bloodstream infections than routine surgical patients [17].

Presence of a chest tube, use of immunosuppressive agents, presence of microbial resistance, length of stay, presence of preexisting infection, percentage change of serum albumin levels, patient disposition, transfusion of 10 or more units of blood, and number of central venous catheters (CVCs) were identified as independent predictors of nosocomial BSI [18].

The most commonly isolated pathogens from blood culture are coagulase-negative *staphylococcus*, *Staphylococcus aureus*, *Enterococcus*, *Candida* spp., *Klebsiella pneumoniae*, and *Pseudomonas aeruginosa*.

Early adequate antimicrobial therapy is an essential determinant of outcome.

Appropriate empirical antibiotic treatment is associated with a significant reduction in fatality in patients with bloodstream infections. After appropriate cultures of blood and catheter samples are done, empirical broad-spectrum i.v. antimicrobial therapy should be initiated as soon as possible. In cases of non-tunneled CVC-related bacteremia and fungemia, the CVC should be removed.

15.7 Intra-abdominal Infections

Hollow viscus injuries (HVIs) are related to significant morbidity and mortality. HVIs are due to both penetrating injury and blunt trauma. They are uncommon in patients with blunt trauma. In these patients a timely diagnosis can be often difficult.

Several mechanisms have been described for bowel injuries occurring after blunt abdominal trauma. Crushing of the bowel segment between the seat belt and vertebra or pelvis posteriorly is the most common mechanism. It results in local lacerations of the bowel wall, mural and mesenteric hematomas, transection of the bowel, localized devascularization, and full-thickness contusions. Devitalization of the areas of contusion may subsequently result in late perforation.

An important determinant of morbidity in patients with HVIs seems to be the time to surgery. Only an expeditious evaluation and diagnosis and prompt surgical intervention can improve the prognosis of these patients [19].

Age, Abdominal Abbreviated Injury Score, the presence of a significant extra-abdominal injury, and a delay of more than 5 h between admission and laparotomy were identified as risk factors for mortality [20].

Generally, the choice of the procedure depends on the anatomical source of infection, on the degree of peritoneal inflammation, on the generalized septic response, and on the patient's general conditions [21].

Also antimicrobial therapy plays an integral role in the management of posttraumatic intra-abdominal infections, especially in critically ill patients. In these patients empirical antimicrobial therapy should be initiated as early as possible.

The major pathogens involved in community-acquired intra-abdominal infection are Enterobacteriaceae, *Streptococcus* spp., and anaerobes (especially *B. fragilis*).

15.8   Surgical Site Infections

Surgical site infections (SSIs) are defined as infections occurring up to 30 days after surgery (or up to 1 year after surgery in patients receiving implants) and affecting either the incision or deep tissue at the operation site. Surgical site infection is the most frequently reported complication in surgical patients, accounting for 14–16 % of all nosocomial infections. In patients undergoing trauma surgery, the incidence of SSIs is higher.

In multivariate analyses, type of trauma (blunt or penetrating), the presence of shock, the number of affected organs, high ISS scores, wound classification, use of prophylactic antibiotics, multiple transfusions, and several surgical procedures have been reported to be risk factors for SSIs in trauma patients [19].

It was found a clear association between contamination of the abdominal cavity (understood as any type of contamination owing to hollow viscus injuries) and SSIs [22].

Undergoing a surgical procedure in the first 24 h after admission offers a protective benefit against the development of SSIs [23].

The causative pathogens of SSIs depend on the type of surgery; the most commonly isolated organisms are *Staphylococcus aureus*, coagulase-negative *staphylococci*, *Enterococcus* spp., and *Escherichia coli*. Numerous patient-related and procedure-related factors influence the risk of SSI in surgical patients, and hence, prevention requires a "bundle" approach, with systematic attention to multiple risk factors, in order to reduce the risk of bacterial contamination and improve the patient's defenses. Good patient preparation, aseptic practice, attention to surgical technique, and antimicrobial prophylaxis are all essential for the prevention of SSIs [24].

References

1. Czaja AS, Rivara FP, Wang J, Koepsell T, Nathens AB, Jurkovich GJ, Mackenzie E (2009) Late outcomes of trauma patients with infections during index hospitalization. J Trauma 67:805–814
2. Glance LG, Stone PW, Mukamel DB, Dick AW (2011) Increases in mortality, length of stay, and cost associated with hospital-acquired infections in trauma patients. Arch Surg 146:794–801
3. Pories SE, Gamelli RL, Mead PB, Goodwin G, Harris F, Vacek P (1991) The epidemiologic features of nosocomial infections in patients with trauma. Arch Surg 126:97–99
4. Jamulitrat S, Narong MN, Thongpiyapoom S (2002) Trauma severity scoring systems as predictors of nosocomial infection. Infect Control Hosp Epidemiol 23:268–273

 5. Serrano PE, Khuder SA, Fath JJ (2010) Obesity as a risk factor for nosocomial infections in trauma patients. J Am Coll Surg 211:61–67
 6. Laird AM, Miller PR, Kilgo PD, Meredith JW, Chang MC (2004) Relationship of early hyperglycemia to mortality in trauma patients. J Trauma 56:1058–1062
 7. Claridge JA, Crabtree TD, Pelletier SJ, Butler K, Sawyer RG, Young JS (2000) Persistent occult hypoperfusion is associated with a significant increase in infection rate and mortality in major trauma patients. J Trauma 48:8–14
 8. Bochicchio GV, Joshi M, Knorr KM, Scalea TM (2001) Impact of nosocomial infections in trauma: does age make a difference? J Trauma 50:612–617
 9. Gannon CJ, Pasquale M, Tracy JK, McCarter RJ, Napolitano LM (2004) Male gender is associated with increased risk for postinjury pneumonia. Shock 21:410–414
10. Andermahr J, Hensler T, Sauerland S, Greb A, Helling HJ, Prokop A, Neugebauer EA, Rehm KE (2003) Risk factors for the development of pneumonia in multiple injured patients. Results of a prospective clinical trial. Unfallchirurg 106:392–397
11. Tejada Artigas A, Bello Dronda S, Chacón Vallés E, Muñoz Marco J, Villuendas Usón MC, Figueras P, Suarez FJ, Hernández A (2001) Risk factors for nosocomial pneumonia in critically ill trauma patients. Crit Care Med 29:304–309
12. Magnotti LJ, Croce MA, Fabian TC (2004) Is ventilator-associated pneumonia in trauma patients an epiphenomenon or a cause of death? Surg Infect (Larchmt) 5:237–242
13. Jones RN (2010) Microbial etiologies of hospital-acquired bacterial pneumonia and ventilator-associated bacterial pneumonia. Clin Infect Dis 51 Suppl 1:S81–S87, 15;171:388–416
14. Alvarez-Lerma F, ICU-Acquired Pneumonia Study Group (1996) Modification of empiric antibiotic treatment in patients with pneumonia acquired in the intensive care unit. Intensive Care Med 22:387–394
15. Monaghan SF, Heffernan DS, Thakkar RK, Reinert SE, Machan JT, Connolly MD, Gregg SC, Kozloff MS, Adams CA Jr, Cioffi WG (2011) The development of a urinary tract infection is associated with increased mortality in trauma patients. J Trauma 71:1569–1574
16. Hooton TM, Bradley SF, Cardenas DD, Colgan R, Geerlings SE, Rice JC, Saint S, Schaeffer AJ, Tambayh PA, Tenke P, Nicolle LE (2010) Infectious Diseases Society of America. Diagnosis, prevention, and treatment of catheter-associated urinary tract infection in adults: 2009

International Clinical Practice Guidelines from the Infectious Diseases Society of America. Clin Infect Dis 50:625–663

17. Wallace WC, Cinat M, Gornick WB, Lekawa ME, Wilson SE (1999) Nosocomial infections in the surgical intensive care unit: a difference between trauma and surgical patients. Am Surg 65:987–990

18. El-Masri MM, Hammad TA, McLeskey SW, Joshi M, Korniewicz DM (2004) Predictors of nosocomial bloodstream infections among critically ill adult trauma patients. Infect Control Hosp Epidemiol 25:656–663

19. Faria GR, Almeida AB, Moreira H, Barbosa E, Correia-da-Silva P, Costa-Maia J (2012) Prognostic factors for traumatic bowel injuries: killing time. World J Surg 36:807–812

20. Malinoski DJ, Patel MS, Yakar DO, Green D, Qureshi F, Inaba K, Brown CV, Salim A (2010) A diagnostic delay of 5 hours increases the risk of death after blunt hollow viscus injury. J Trauma 69:84–87

21. Sartelli M, Viale P, Koike K, Pea F, Tumietto F, van Goor H, Guercioni G, Nespoli A, Tranà C, Catena F, Ansaloni L, Leppaniemi A, Biffl W, Moore FA, Poggetti R, Pinna AD, Moore EE (2011) WSES consensus conference: guidelines for first-line management of intra-abdominal infections. World J Emerg Surg 6:2

22. Morales CH, Escobar RM, Villegas MI, Castaño A, Trujillo J (2011) Surgical site infection in abdominal trauma patients: risk prediction and performance of the NNIS and SENIC indexes. Can J Surg 54:17–24

23. Cheadle WG (2006) Risk factors for surgical site infection. Surg Infect (Larchmt) 7 Suppl 1:S7–S11

24. Owens CD, Stoessel K (2008) Surgical site infections: epidemiology, microbiology and prevention. J Hosp Infect 70(Suppl 2):3–10

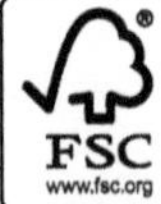

MIX
Papier aus verantwortungsvollen Quellen
Paper from responsible sources
FSC® C105338

If you have any concerns about our products,
you can contact us on
ProductSafety@springernature.com

In case Publisher is established outside the EU,
the EU authorized representative is:
Springer Nature Customer Service Center GmbH
Europaplatz 3, 69115 Heidelberg, Germany

Printed by Libri Plureos GmbH
in Hamburg, Germany